NURSING PHOTOBOOK

Using Monitors

NURSING80 BOOKS
INTERMED COMMUNICATIONS, INC.
HORSHAM, PENNSYLVANIA

Nursing80 Books
NURSING PHOTOBOOK™ Series
PUBLISHER
Eugene W. Jackson

EDITORIAL DIRECTOR
Jean Robinson

CLINICAL DIRECTOR
Barbara McVan, RN

ART DIRECTOR
Daniel Panachyda

MANUFACTURING DIRECTOR
Bernard Haas

**Intermed Communications
Book Division**
DIRECTOR
John L. Rikhoff

DIRECTOR, RESEARCH
Elizabeth O'Brien

DIRECTOR, PRODUCTION AND PURCHASING
Bacil Guiley

Staff for this volume
BOOK EDITOR
Richard Samuel West

CLINICAL EDITOR
Helene Ritting Nawrocki, RN

ASSOCIATE EDITOR
Katherine W. Carey

PHOTOGRAPHER
Paul A. Cohen

DESIGNERS
Lisa A. Gilde
Linda A. Jovinelly
Carol Stickles

EDITORIAL/GRAPHIC COORDINATOR
Doreen K. Stowers

CLINICAL/GRAPHIC COORDINATOR
Evelyn M. James

COPY EDITOR
Barbara Hodgson

COPY ASSISTANT
David Beverage

EDITORIAL ASSISTANT
Cynthia A. Lotz

PHOTOGRAPHY ASSISTANT
Thomas Staudenmayer

DARKROOM ASSISTANT
Gary Donnelly

ART PRODUCTION MANAGER
Wilbur D. Davidson

ART ASSISTANTS
Lorraine Carbo   Sandra Simms
Darcy Feralio   Louise Stamper
Diane Fox   Joan Walsh
Robert Perry   Ron Yablon

RESEARCHER
Vonda Heller

TYPOGRAPHY MANAGER
David C. Kosten

ASSISTANT TO THE
TYPOGRAPHY MANAGER
David Davenport

TYPOGRAPHY ASSISTANTS
Ethel Halle
Diane Paluba

PRODUCTION MANAGER
Robert L. Dean, Jr.

ASSISTANT PRODUCTION MANAGER
Deborah C. Meiris

PRODUCTION ASSISTANT
M. Eileen Hunsicker

ILLUSTRATORS
Jack Crane   Gerald Kolpan
Jean Gardner   Cynthia Mason
Tom Hallman   Kim Milnazik
Tom Herbert   Henry Rothman
Robert Jackson   Bud Yingling

SERIES GRAPHIC DESIGNER
John C. Isely

COVER PHOTO
Seymour Mednick

**Clinical consultants
for this volume**
Judith Ann Bailey, RN, BSN, MBA
Nurse Coordinator
Regional Trauma Center, University Hospital
University of California Medical Center
San Diego, California

Albert F. Mutton, Jr., BS, MS, RCPT
Instructor, Respiratory Therapy Technology
Forsyth Technical Institute
Winston-Salem, North Carolina

Library of Congress Cataloging in Publication Data

Main entry under title:

Using monitors.

  (Nursing photobook)
  Bibliography: p.
  Includes index.
  1. Patient monitoring.   2. Nursing.
I. Intermed Communications, Inc.
  [DNLM: 1. Monitoring, Physiologic—Instrumentation—
  Nursing texts.
  WY150 U85]
RT48.U84   610.73   80-20948
ISBN 0-916730-26-3

Contents

Contributors

Donna R. Ambrogi was a staff nurse in the neurosensory intensive care unit at Thomas Jefferson University Hospital in Philadelphia. A graduate of Thomas Jefferson University Hospital School of Nursing, she's currently a BSN candidate at the University of San Francisco.

F. Patrick Ausband is vice president, nursing service (director of nursing) at Lexington (N.C.) Memorial Hospital. Formerly, he was educational coordinator for respiratory care service at Forsyth Memorial Hospital in Winston-Salem, N.C. After earning his ADN at Davidson County Community College in Lexington, he received his BSN from Winston-Salem State University. A member of the National Board for Respiratory Therapy, Mr. Ausband is a certified respiratory therapy technician.

Judith Ann Bailey, an adviser for this PHOTOBOOK, is nurse coordinator for the Regional Trauma Center, University of California Medical Center, San Diego. She received her BSN from San Diego State College and her MBA from National University, also in San Diego.

Bonnie Berk, a certified childbirth educator, is a clinical obstetrics/gynecology instructor at St. Agnes Hospital in Philadelphia. Formerly, she was a delivery room staff nurse at Pennsylvania Hospital, also in Philadelphia. A graduate of Albert Einstein Medical Center School of Nursing (Philadelphia), she's currently a BS candidate in health education at Temple University, also in Philadelphia.

Kathleen Geraghty Burke is a medical/surgical instructor at Episcopal Hospital in Philadelphia. Formerly, she was an intensive care unit primary nurse at Albert Einstein Medical Center, also in Philadelphia. She's a graduate of Pennsylvania State University in University Park.

Mary G. Cooney is intensive care unit head nurse at Albert Einstein Medical Center in Philadelphia. She received her nursing diploma from Middlesex County College, Edison, N.J.

Linda J. Corcoran is the assistant head nurse in charge of orientation in the infant intensive care unit at Children's Hospital of Philadelphia. She earned her BSN from Villanova (Pa.) University.

Cindy Dalsey is an intensive care unit staff nurse at Albert Einstein Medical Center in Philadelphia. She earned her nursing diploma from the Community Medical Center School of Nursing in Scranton, Pa.

Ann Elsden is cardiac care unit head nurse at Toronto Western Hospital, where she also teaches cardiac monitoring and telemetry to staff nurses. For 5 years, at Toronto Western Hospital, she was clinical instructor for the postgraduate coronary care program (clinical component) for Humber College of Applied Arts and Technology. Ms. Elsden is a graduate of Queen Elizabeth Hospital School of Nursing in Montreal.

Susan T. Hill, a certified childbirth educator, was perinatal testing nurse and coordinator of the childbirth education program at Pennsylvania Hospital in Philadelphia. Currently, she's an MSN candidate in nurse midwifery at the University of Pennsylvania, also in Philadelphia. Ms. Hill earned her diploma from the Hospital of the University of Pennsylvania School of Nursing, and her BSN from Gwynedd-Mercy College in Gwynedd Valley, Pa.

Janet M. McMenamin, a recovery room nurse at Albert Einstein Medical Center, Philadelphia, was formerly assistant head nurse, intensive care unit, Albert Einstein Medical Center. A graduate of D'Youville College in Buffalo, N.Y., she's currently a MSN candidate at the University of Pennsylvania in Philadelphia.

Albert F. Mutton, Jr., also an adviser for this PHOTOBOOK, is an instructor of respiratory therapy technology at Forsyth Technical Institute in Winston-Salem, N.C. He received his BS and MS degrees from East Tennessee State University in Johnson City. A member of the National Society of Cardiopulmonary Technology, he's a registered cardiopulmonary technologist.

Julia A. Pelensky, a graduate of Villanova (Pa.) University, is a cardiovascular nurse at Albert Einstein Medical Center in Philadelphia.

Claire J. Pudlinski is an intensive care unit staff nurse at Albert Einstein Medical Center in Philadelphia. A graduate of the Albert Einstein Medical Center School of Nursing, she's currently a BSN candidate at Gwynedd-Mercy College, Gwynedd Valley, Pa.

Leslie K. Sampson is patient care coordinator for the intensive care unit, recovery room, and emergency unit at Albert Einstein Medical Center in Philadelphia. A graduate of Philadelphia General Hospital School of Nursing, Mr. Sampson is currently a BSN candidate at LaSalle College, Philadelphia.

Introduction

Using monitors. Does the thought scare you? If it does, then you're like most nurses. Working with monitors challenges even the most experienced of us. After all, you must first complete complex procedures to initiate monitoring, and then, be ready in case anything goes wrong.

Every day, doctors rely on the special skills of nurses, particularly when monitors are involved. In some hospitals, the nurse is the only health-care professional trained to use monitors. That's why knowing how to operate the equipment is so important. That's also why you need this unique PHOTOBOOK. It's the first book that shows and explains exactly how to work every major type of monitor. And it does so in the style that PHOTOBOOKS are noted for: with step-by-step photostories; easy-to-understand text; troubleshooting charts on common equipment problems; detailed anatomical illustrations; and helpful nursing tips.

To make sure you never forget your biggest responsibility—your patient's well-being—we've opened this PHOTOBOOK with a section on patient care. Next, we explore the latest methods for measuring intracranial pressure. In this section, you'll learn about some of the most sensitive monitoring equipment available: the subarachnoid screw, the ventricular catheter, and the epidural sensor.

In Section 3, we show you how to operate cardiac monitors: hardwire, telemetry, and Holter. On these pages, you'll find charts that make EKG interpretation easier.

Measuring hemodynamic pressure won't be nearly as difficult after you read Section 4. Photostories and charts in this section will make you an expert on arterial lines, pulmonary artery lines, and left atrial lines.

We introduce you to some of the most innovative monitors around today in the last two sections. For example, in the section on measuring respiratory functions, you'll learn the skills necessary to cope with the mass spectrometer, the transcutaneous pO_2 monitor, and the apnea monitor. You'll be coached on how to prepare the family who must care for an infant on an apnea monitor. In addition, you can copy the special home care aid we've included to use in your patient teaching.

Finally, in Section 6, we make the complicated whys and hows of fetal monitoring easy to understand. In those pages, you'll learn how to initiate noninvasive methods and how to assist the doctor with invasive methods.

If you think about it, monitors are only a worry when you don't know how to operate them. But, with this unique PHOTOBOOK, you can learn all you need to know. Consider this book a valuable tool. Let it help you meet—and overcome—the challenge of using monitors.

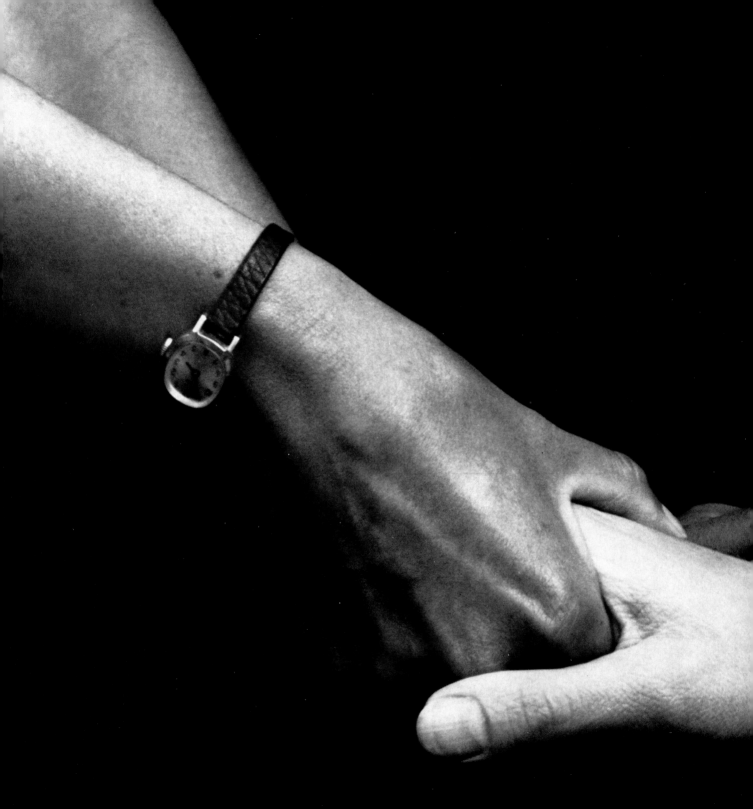

Managing Patient Care

Guidelines and precautions

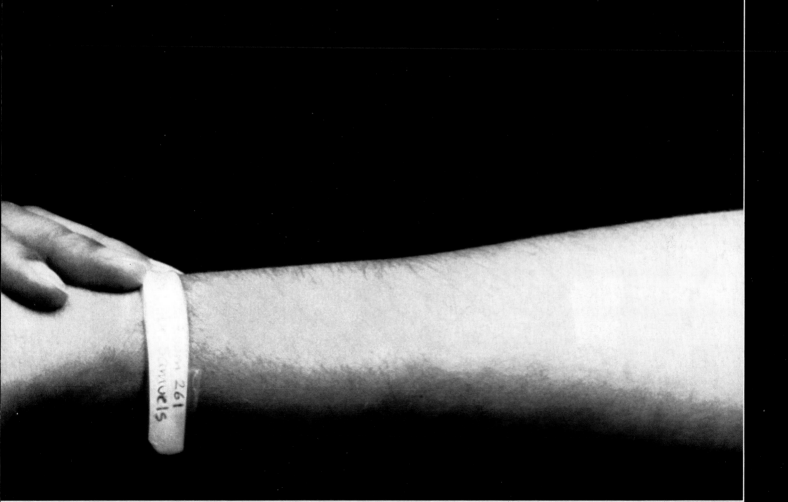

Guidelines and precautions

What do many nurses think is the most challenging aspect of working with monitors? Learning proper setup techniques? Troubleshooting equipment problems effectively? Reading printouts accurately?

None of these. The *patient* being monitored, not the monitor itself, poses the greatest challenge. Why? Because when you work with monitors, you'll find it's so easy to be-come wrapped up managing the equipment that you forget the patient's even there.

How can you provide top-notch patient care *and* expert monitoring at the same time? The goal is a difficult one, but achieving it will make you more than just a competent nurse. You'll be indispensable to both the hospital and your patients. Always remember: As impor-tant as technical proficiency is, patient care must never be over-looked.

Read the next few pages care-fully, and refer to them occasion-ally. If you always remember the patient's needs and still become a monitor expert, you'll have success-fully met the biggest challenge of using monitors.

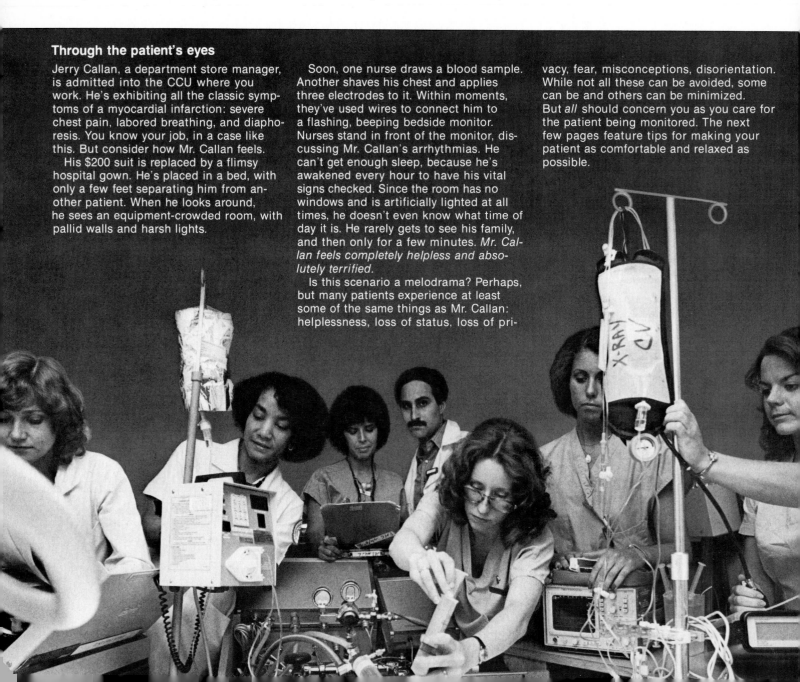

Through the patient's eyes

Jerry Callan, a department store manager, is admitted into the CCU where you work. He's exhibiting all the classic symp-toms of a myocardial infarction: severe chest pain, labored breathing, and diapho-resis. You know your job, in a case like this. But consider how Mr. Callan feels.

His $200 suit is replaced by a flimsy hospital gown. He's placed in a bed, with only a few feet separating him from an-other patient. When he looks around, he sees an equipment-crowded room, with pallid walls and harsh lights.

Soon, one nurse draws a blood sample. Another shaves his chest and applies three electrodes to it. Within moments, they've used wires to connect him to a flashing, beeping bedside monitor. Nurses stand in front of the monitor, dis-cussing Mr. Callan's arrhythmias. He can't get enough sleep, because he's awakened every hour to have his vital signs checked. Since the room has no windows and is artificially lighted at all times, he doesn't even know what time of day it is. He rarely gets to see his family, and then only for a few minutes. *Mr. Cal-lan feels completely helpless and abso-lutely terrified.*

Is this scenario a melodrama? Perhaps, but many patients experience at least some of the same things as Mr. Callan: helplessness, loss of status, loss of pri-vacy, fear, misconceptions, disorientation. While not all these can be avoided, some can be and others can be minimized. But *all* should concern you as you care for the patient being monitored. The next few pages feature tips for making your patient as comfortable and relaxed as possible.

Patient first, monitor second

Patient care can be a difficult skill to master. It requires enormous amounts of time, perseverence, empathy, and energy—things in great demand in all hospitals. But when the patient needs monitoring, the requirements are even greater. You must set up and maintain sophisticated equipment, without forgetting or ignoring your patient. Here are some guidelines to help you meet her physical—and emotional—needs:

Explain the monitoring procedure to her step by step, so she knows what to expect. Tell her why she's being monitored and how it'll help. Probe what she knows about monitoring, then clear up any misconceptions. For example, is she afraid the alarm will go off when she moves? Does she think she'll get a shock from the electrodes? Anticipate such concerns and relieve her anxieties.

Find out how she feels about being hospitalized. For example, does she resent the lack of privacy, the constant interruptions, the impersonal rooms, and the restrictions on visitors? Once you've identified what's making her unhappy, do your best to minimize it. If possible, adjust your scheduling to accommodate her need. Encourage family members to bring personal items from home. Ask the doctor to relax some of the visiting restrictions. If you can't do anything to change the situation, explain why. Remember, sharing your patient's concerns will enhance your rapport with her.

As monitoring progresses, don't let the monitor become more important to you than your patient. *When you enter her room, greet her first and attend to her needs before you go to the monitor.* Don't discuss her condition with others at her bedside unless you include her in the discussions, too. If the monitor sounds an alarm, always check the patient first, then the equipment. For details on how to cope with these responsibilities on your busy schedule, read the following pages.

Keep in mind that monitors are only a *tool* in nursing. They don't replace the attention and care you give a patient, and never will. A nurse's keen observations can be the best monitor of a patient's progress.

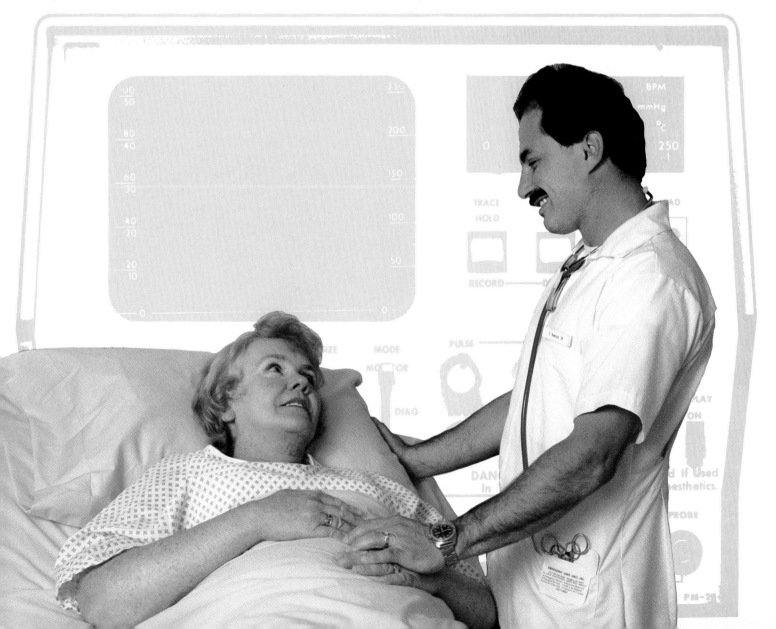

Guidelines and precautions

Minimizing electrical hazards

Did you know that, each year, thousands of people are electrocuted by monitoring equipment? The number of fatalities is staggering, but what's worse is that the vast majority of these deaths can be avoided by observation of simple, yet crucial, grounding precautions.

Do you know these precautions? Implement the following to safeguard yourself and your patient:
• Don't use two-pronged plugs or three-way outlet adapters. All monitors should feature three-pronged, grounded plugs and should be inserted directly into a wall outlet.
• Don't use equipment that has a frayed or cracked electrical cord. Don't place a cord where it can be accidentally severed or get wet.
• Don't use any equipment without first attaching it to a common ground, using a three-wire circuit. Never ground equipment to a water pipe or a common cable.
• Don't use equipment that malfunctions in any way; for example, equipment that sparks, smokes, overheats, or issues mild shocks. If a monitor does any of these while it's connected to the patient, disconnect it immediately and replace it. If it cannot be replaced quickly, notify the doctor. To guard against malfunction, make sure all monitors are inspected regularly.
• Don't place wet items—especially beverages or damp towels—on top of a monitor or other electrical equipment. If liquid is spilled or seeps into a room with electrical equipment, make sure you wipe it up immediately.

Through the nurse's eyes

You know the patient comes first. You've always known that. The hard part is *keeping* the patient first when you're pressed for time. Picture this:

Two of your coworkers in the ICU call in sick. A new I.V. pump is being used for the first time, and no one is comfortable with it. The wife of one patient has called for the third time this morning to ask about her husband. One of the cardiac monitors is malfunctioning. And the chief of staff is complaining that the jugular line setup he ordered isn't ready. To make matters worse, at any moment you may have to make snap decisions and initiate intervention that could dramatically affect your patients' conditions. How are you going to find time to talk to and comfort your patients?

Sounds like a cruel joke? You bet it does. Theoretically, the patient comes first, but under the stress of the ICU, that doesn't always happen. What can you do about it?

Say you're faced with taking hourly blood pressure readings, measuring urine output, and giving medications for not one, but *four* patients. Don't let the burden of future tasks weigh on your mind. As you go about your work, explain what you're doing to each patient, touch his hand occasionally, and ask concerned questions. Talking with him while you work takes no more time. Moreover, if it serves to lessen some of his anxiety, he may not need a sedative later. Then you'll have *saved* time—as well as helped him—by not having to give him an injection.

You can probably suggest many other situations like this one, where you can use time spent on a mechanical task to enhance your patient care. Extra effort's required to conscientiously change your habits, but if your patient benefits, it's effort well spent.

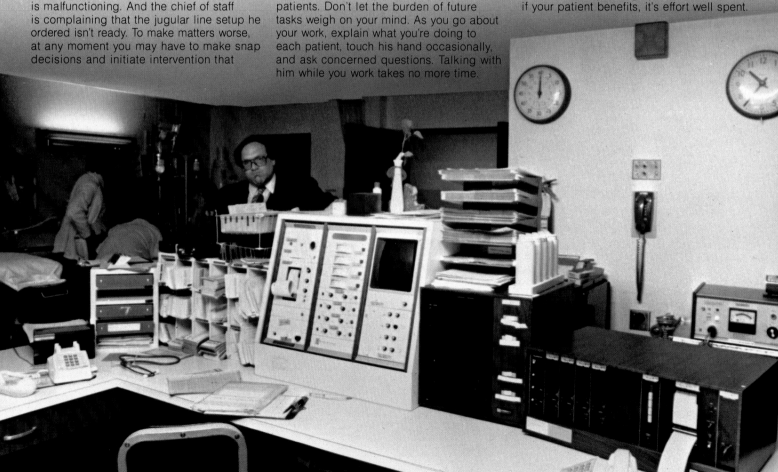

Troubleshooting monitors: A systematic method

You're working in a CCU unit dispensing medication when a monitor alarm sounds. Your natural reaction is to look toward where the sound is coming from: the monitor. But fight that reaction. Even if you suspect that the monitor's malfunctioning—and the alarm's not an indication that the patient's condition is deteriorating—*don't take any chances*. First, determine without question that your patient doesn't need attention. Then, look at the equipment.

Here's a simple, systematic method for troubleshooting: Begin with the patient, and proceed outward to the monitor. This method not only safeguards your patient's health, but it eliminates time-wasting guesswork by drawing attention to the most likely problems first.

Use this checklist:
1. Check patient.
2. Check insertion site or electrode site.
3. Check tubing or lead wire.
4. Check connections to monitor.
5. Check monitor.
6. Check connection to electrical outlet.

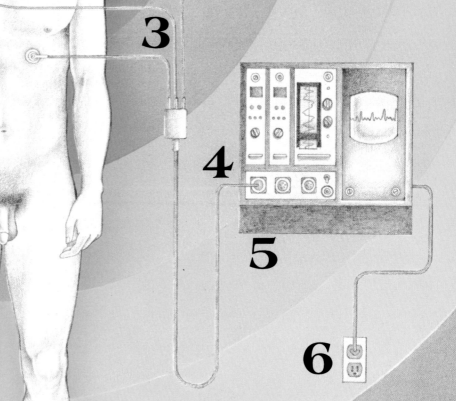

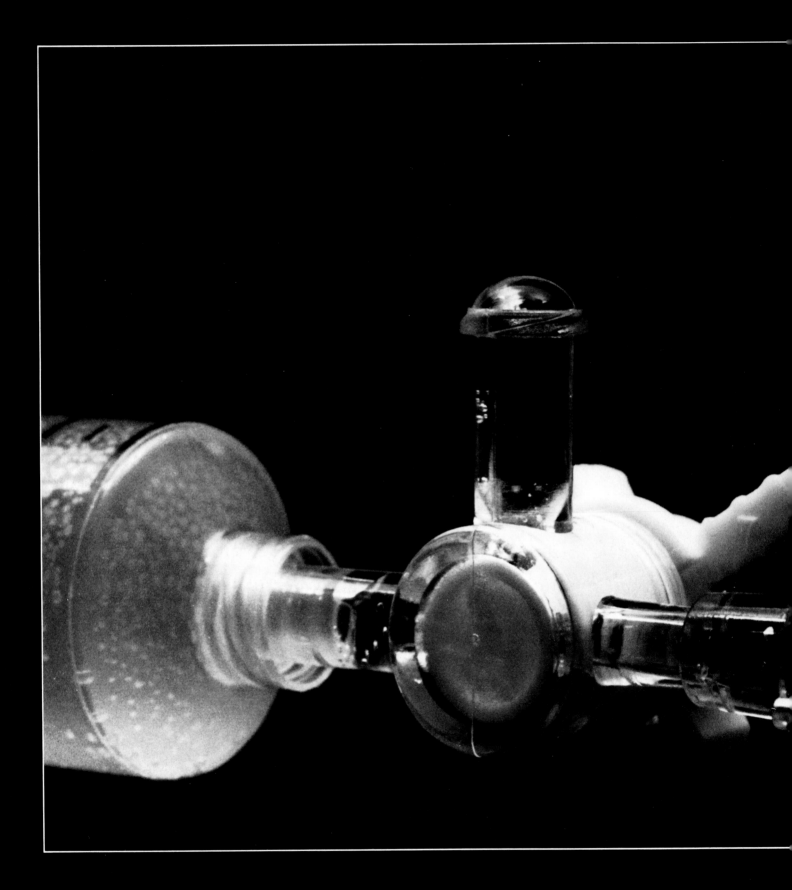

Measuring Intracranial Pressure

Pressure monitoring basics

Intracranial monitors

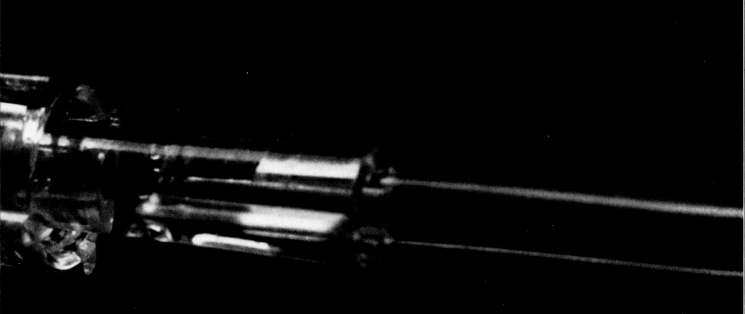

Pressure monitoring basics

Most invasive pressure monitoring systems, including most of those measuring intracranial pressure (ICP), consist of a monitor, a pressure transducer, and a fluid-filled line to the patient. Chances are, you've used this type of system before. But did you really understand how it works?

On the following pages, we'll review the basics: balancing and calibrating the transducer, and calibrating the monitor. Because of the variety of equipment available, we'll feature several types of monitors and transducers. With this background, you'll be ready to set up any of these pressure monitoring systems: intracranial, hemodynamic, or uterine.

Understanding transducers

You'll use pressure transducers during intracranial pressure (ICP) monitoring (with a subarachnoid screw or ventricular catheter), hemodynamic monitoring, and some types of uterine monitoring. Do you know how transducers work? If not, examine these photos.

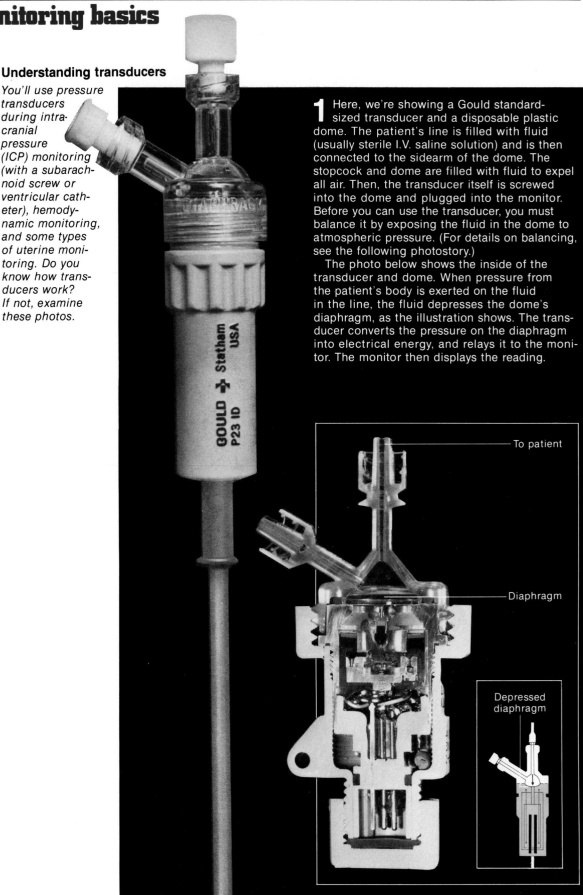

1 Here, we're showing a Gould standard-sized transducer and a disposable plastic dome. The patient's line is filled with fluid (usually sterile I.V. saline solution) and is then connected to the sidearm of the dome. The stopcock and dome are filled with fluid to expel all air. Then, the transducer itself is screwed into the dome and plugged into the monitor. Before you can use the transducer, you must balance it by exposing the fluid in the dome to atmospheric pressure. (For details on balancing, see the following photostory.)

The photo below shows the inside of the transducer and dome. When pressure from the patient's body is exerted on the fluid in the line, the fluid depresses the dome's diaphragm, as the illustration shows. The transducer converts the pressure on the diaphragm into electrical energy, and relays it to the monitor. The monitor then displays the reading.

To patient

Diaphragm

Depressed diaphragm

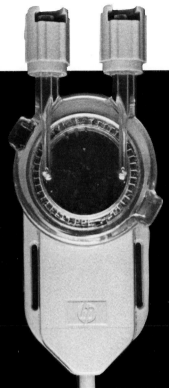

2 This is a Hewlett-Packard quartz transducer, with a disposable plastic dome in place. Because its diaphragm is a resilient quartz plate, this transducer can withstand very high pressure without damage. To set up this transducer, you'll use a procedure similar to the one for a standard-sized transducer. (Check the operator's manual for complete instructions.)

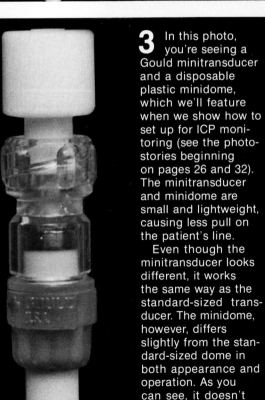

3 In this photo, you're seeing a Gould minitransducer and a disposable plastic minidome, which we'll feature when we show how to set up for ICP monitoring (see the photostories beginning on pages 26 and 32). The minitransducer and minidome are small and lightweight, causing less pull on the patient's line.

Even though the minitransducer looks different, it works the same way as the standard-sized transducer. The minidome, however, differs slightly from the standard-sized dome in both appearance and operation. As you can see, it doesn't have a sidearm. When you balance this transducer, you must open a *stopcock port* to air.

Balancing a standard-sized transducer

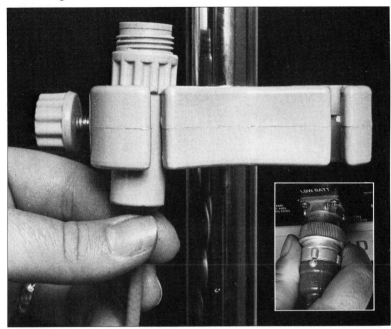

1 *How can you be sure that your pressure readings are accurate? The first step is to balance (or zero) the transducer to atmospheric pressure. By balancing, you establish atmospheric pressure as the baseline for your patient's pressure readings. In effect, you prevent atmospheric pressure from affecting the patient's pressure readings.*

You can balance the transducer before or after you connect the system to the patient. The procedures are the same, except that the dome will be air-filled if you balance the transducer before you connect the system, and fluid-filled if you balance the transducer afterward.

This photostory will show you how to balance a standard-sized transducer. For details on how to balance a minitransducer, turn to page 31.

First, mount the transducer on an I.V. pole with a transducer holder. Then, plug it into the monitor, as the inset shows. Turn on the monitor. (The monitor and transducer need 10 to 15 minutes to warm up.)

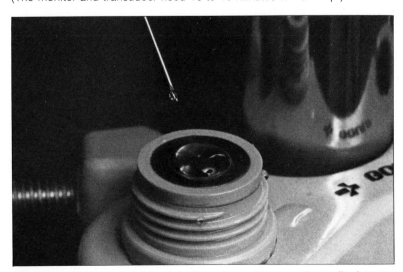

2 Next, put several drops of sterile water on the transducer diaphragm. *Note:* Don't use tap water. It contains impurities that may damage the transducer diaphragm.

Pressure monitoring basics

Balancing a standard-sized transducer continued

3 Now, securely screw the dome onto the transducer.

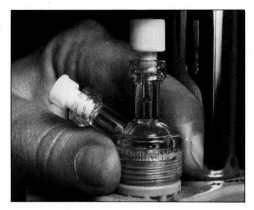

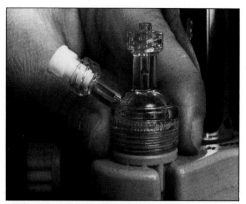

5 Uncap the dome's upright arm (balancing port). Now, the transducer's diaphragm is exposed to atmospheric pressure.

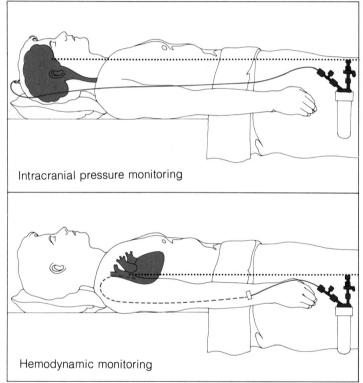

Intracranial pressure monitoring

Hemodynamic monitoring

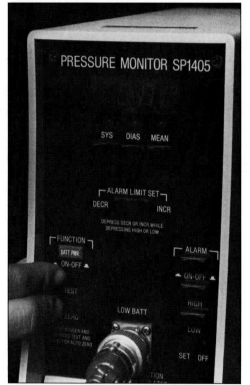

6 If your monitor has an automatic ZERO button, like the one shown here, depress it. Then, take a look at the reading on the monitor. It will automatically read zero. Now, the transducer's balanced to atmospheric pressure.

Note: If your monitor *doesn't* have an automatic ZERO button, balance the transducer manually. To do this, turn the ZERO knob on the monitor until the reading is zero.

4 As you know, to balance the transducer you must open one of the dome's arms to atmospheric pressure. When you use a standard-sized dome, choose the upright arm as your balancing port, because it's easier than the sidearm to level correctly.

How do you level it? Position the top of the balancing port—*not* the transducer itself—so it's level with the patient's pressure source (the part of his body you're monitoring).

Take a look at the above illustrations. When you're doing intracranial pressure (ICP) monitoring, the pressure source is the foramen of Monro. Therefore, position the top of the balancing port level with a point between the end of the patient's eyebrow and the tragus of his ear. When you're doing hemodynamic monitoring, position the balancing port level with the patient's right atrium.

Remember to maintain the balancing port at the proper level throughout monitoring. If the patient moves, reposition and rebalance the transducer. For each inch off the proper level, you can expect a 2 mm Hg error in the pressure reading.

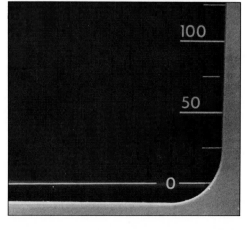

7 Now, look at the oscilloscope screen. When the transducer's balanced, you'll see a flat wave at zero, as shown here.

Finally, cap the balancing port. Now you're ready to calibrate the monitor with the transducer. To learn how, read on.

How to calibrate the monitor with the transducer

Before you begin monitoring your patient's pressure, make sure the monitor will interpret the transducer's signal correctly. To do this, calibrate the monitor to the transducer.

Begin by balancing the transducer, as shown on the preceding pages. Don't forget to cap the balancing port. (Leave the line open between the monitor and the transducer, and closed to the patient.)

Your next step depends on the type of monitor you're using. (Check the operator's manual for complete instructions.) Most likely, the monitor can be calibrated by one of these three procedures: cal factor, electric cal, or pre-cal. The following photos show how these calibration methods differ.

Important: The calibration procedures described below ensure that the monitor's reading corresponds to the transducer's sensitivity. But they *don't* ensure that the pressure reading itself is accurate. That's why you must periodically use a mercury sphygmomanometer to apply a known pressure to the transducer, and calibrate the monitor to that pressure. To do this correctly, simply follow the procedure shown on page 18.

Cal factor

Some monitors, like the Electronics for Medicine (E for M) monitor shown here, will operate with several types of transducers. But before you can calibrate the monitor with the transducer, you must know the transducer's cal factor. If the cal factor's not marked on the transducer, you can find it by testing the transducer with a mercury sphygmomanometer (see page 18). Then, when you've found the cal factor, follow these steps:

[Inset 1] Depress the BALANCE button, as shown here. If the transducer's balanced properly, you'll get a zero reading. Release the BALANCE button.

[Inset 2] Next, depress the CALIBRATE button and hold it.

[Inset 3] Using a screwdriver, turn the screw next to the CALIBRATE button until the digital reading equals the transducer's cal factor. Now the transducer and monitor are calibrated with each other.

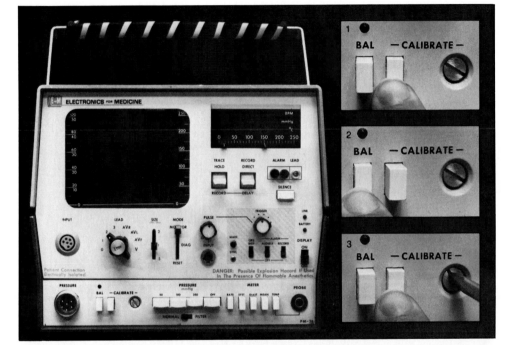

Electric cal

This is a Hewlett-Packard monitor. Unlike the E for M monitor shown above, this monitor determines the transducer's cal factor electronically. But you can't use any type of transducer—just the special Hewlett-Packard transducer made for this monitor.

To calibrate this system, use the electric cal method:

[Inset 1] Depress the ZERO button on the monitor.

[Inset 2] Now, depress the TEST/CAL button.

[Inset 3] Finally, turn the SENSITIVITY knob until the digital reading is 100 mm Hg. For this particular monitor, consider a 100 mm Hg reading a sure indication that the monitor and the transducer are calibrated to each other.

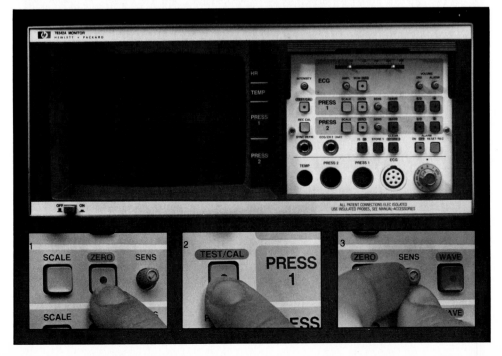

Pressure monitoring basics

How to calibrate the monitor with the transducer *continued*

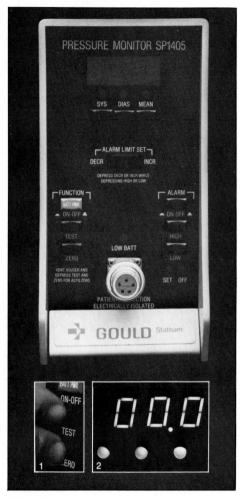

Pre-cal

Like the Hewlett-Packard monitor shown on the preceding page, this Gould monitor requires a specially made transducer to work. Because the monitor and transducer are already calibrated with each other, all you have to do is test them to make sure they're working properly. Here's how:
[Inset 1] Depress the TEST button and ZERO button simultaneously, and hold them.
[Inset 2] Observe the digital reading, which will be zero if the equipment's working properly.

If the digital reading isn't zero, check the monitor and transducer to make sure they've had a chance to warm up. If they have, and the reading still isn't zero, replace the monitor and call the manufacturer for service. Don't try to calibrate the equipment yourself.

Important: Routinely balance and calibrate each transducer and monitor at least once every 4 hours for intracranial pressure lines; every 8 hours for hemodynamic and uterine lines.

Testing the transducer with a mercury sphygmomanometer

You've just balanced your transducer, following the guidelines shown on page 16. Are the pressure readings accurate? Not necessarily. With prolonged use, all transducers lose some sensitivity and become less accurate. The exact degree of inaccuracy is called the cal factor. *To compensate for the cal factor, you must adjust the monitor.*

How do you determine a transducer's cal factor? First, obtain an ordinary mercury sphygmomanometer and a plastic Y-connector. After the transducer and monitor have warmed up, follow these steps.

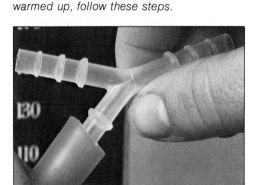

1 Remove the cuff from the mercury sphygmomanometer. Attach the sphygmomanometer's rubber tubing to one arm of the Y-connector, as shown here.

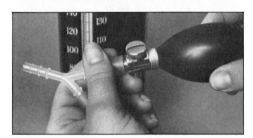

2 Then, attach the sphygmomanometer's bulb to the other arm of the Y-connector.

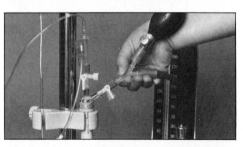

3 Using a stopcock, connect the foot of the Y-connector to one arm of the transducer dome; then, open the stopcock between the Y-connector and the dome. Make sure the stopcock on the *other* arm of the dome is off to the transducer.

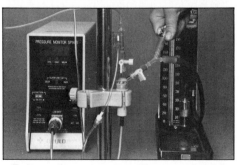

4 If the sphygmomanometer's mercury column reads zero, pump up the sphygmomanometer until the column reaches 200 mm Hg. This applies 200 mm Hg of pressure to the transducer's diaphragm. Now, look at the monitor's digital reading. If the transducer's lost some sensitivity (which is likely), the digital reading *won't* equal 200 mm Hg. Adjust the CAL or SENS (sensitivity control) button until it does.

Release the pressure on the mercury sphygmomanometer, and wait for the mercury column to return to zero. Now, press the CAL button again. The number displayed by the digital reading is the cal factor.

Mark the cal factor on a piece of tape, and fasten the tape to the transducer's cable for easy reference. However, don't forget to recheck the cal factor periodically. Transducers are fragile instruments, and their cal factors may change.

You'll use the cal factor to calibrate the transducer with some types of monitors. For more details, review page 17.

Selecting an oscilloscope range

Before you calibrate the oscilloscope, select a pressure range. Most oscilloscopes provide at least two choices: 100 mm Hg or 200 mm Hg. Some oscilloscopes have more.

The range indicates the highest pressure the oscilloscope will measure. The amplitude of the pressure you're monitoring will determine your selection. Choose a low range for low amplitude pressures (for example, central venous pressure [CVP] or left atrial pressure); a high range for high amplitude pressures (for example, arterial blood pressure, unless the patient's hypotensive). Use the monitor's digital reading as a guide.

Why is range selection important? Suppose you're monitoring right atrial CVP. If the range is set at 200 mm Hg, the waveform will be so small that you won't be able to see it clearly. However, suppose you're monitoring high arterial blood pressure. If the range is set at 100 mm Hg or lower, the waveform will be too big to fit on the screen. In either case, adjust the monitor's pressure range knob so the waveform is clearly—and completely—visible.

How to balance and calibrate an oscilloscope

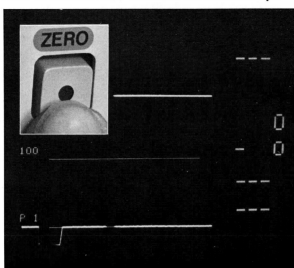

1 *If your monitor includes an oscilloscope, you must balance and calibrate it, too. Here's how:*

First, open the transducer's balancing port to air. Then, press the monitor's ZERO button (see inset). When the baseline registers zero, as shown on this oscilloscope, close the balancing port.

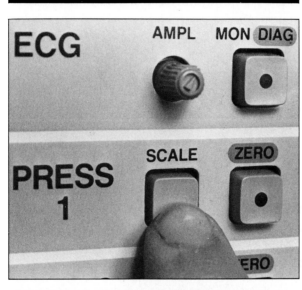

2 Next, select a pressure range by pressing the SCALE button. For guidelines on range selection, see the left side of this page. If you're monitoring arterial blood pressure for a hypotensive patient, for example, you'll probably select the 100 mm Hg range.

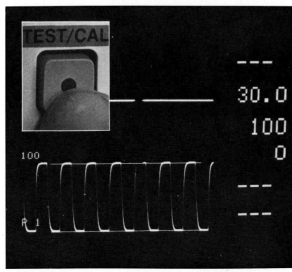

3 Depress the TEST/CAL button, as shown in the inset. On the oscilloscope screen, you'll see a waveform like the one shown here. If the top of the waveform doesn't rise to 100 mm Hg, adjust the sensitivity control knob until it does.

Note: If your oscilloscope has several channels, you must balance and calibrate each one.

How to calibrate a recorder

Most likely, you can connect the monitor to a recorder to get readout strips. But before you use the recorder, calibrate it to the monitor. (Since the calibrating procedure may vary slightly with some models, read your operator's manual carefully before beginning.)

First, load the recorder with recorder paper, according to the operator's instructions. Turn on the recorder to a slow speed. Then, place the recorder's stylus on the zero line of the paper. The stylus will draw a flat baseline at zero.

On the left side of this page, you learned how to select a pressure range for the oscilloscope. Use this pressure range as a guide when you calibrate the recorder. For example, suppose the pressure range is 200 mm Hg. To calibrate the recorder to the monitor, depress the *monitor's* TEST/CAL button and hold it. Then, adjust the *recorder's* GAIN knob until the baseline rises to 200 mm Hg on the recorder paper. Then, release the TEST/CAL button. Now the recorder's calibrated to the monitor.

Intracranial monitors

Almost every health-care professional recognizes the danger signs of increased intracranial pressure (ICP): a change in the patient's level of consciousness; headache; vomiting; pupillary changes; or deterioration of motor function. So why monitor ICP invasively and expose your patient to unnecessary risks?

The reason's simple: These clinical danger signs are notoriously unreliable and may suggest any number of conditions. But even when they do signal an ICP rise, they may appear long after the brain's suffered serious damage.

How does ICP monitoring help? By buying time. When you continuously monitor a patient's ICP, you're aware of the slightest change in ICP as soon as it occurs. The doctor can then begin therapy to lower the ICP before it reaches a dangerous level.

How much do you know about the three basic ICP monitoring systems? Can you interpret waveforms? Troubleshoot problems? Tailor your nursing care to the patient's special needs? The following pages will give you the information you need to monitor ICP accurately.

Reviewing the brain's anatomy

If you're like most nurses, you're a little rusty when it comes to the brain's anatomy and physiology. To review, examine these illustrations. They'll help you understand the specifics of intracranial pressure (ICP) monitoring.

As you can see in the illustration below, the largest part of the brain is the cerebrum, which is divided into the right and the left hemispheres. The cerebellum lies beneath the cerebrum, in the back of the skull. The pons and medulla—the main sections of the brain stem—lie beneath the cerebrum, in front of the cerebellum.

As the cross section on the opposite page shows, the brain's enveloped by three meninges, or membranes, which help protect the brain from shock and infection: the pia mater, the arachnoid, and the dura mater. The narrow subarachnoid space between the arachnoid and the pia mater contains cerebrospinal fluid (CSF). If necessary, the doctor may place a subarachnoid screw into this space to measure your patient's ICP.

Portions of the dura mater—the falx cerebri and the tentorium—extend into the brain's fissures. The falx cerebri lies in the longitudinal fissure, and separates the right and left hemi-spheres of the brain. The tentorium lies in the transverse fissure, and separates the cerebrum and cerebellum.

Each of the brain's four ventricles contains clusters of capillaries, called choroid plexus. These capillaries produce approximately 21 ml of CSF per hour. From the ventricles, CSF circulates as shown in the large illustration on the opposite page, cushioning the brain from injury and transporting wastes and nutrients. Eventually, it's absorbed in the brain's venous sinuses—primarily the superior sagittal sinus—through the arachnoid villi, which are vascular protrusions of the arachnoid. In a healthy adult, the circulating volume of cerebrospinal fluid is 100 to 150 ml.

The skull has many openings, or foramina, that permit nerves and blood vessels to reach the brain. These foramina also allow CSF to circulate around the spinal cord and brain.

As you can see in the illustration below, two of the larger foramina are the tentorial notch and the foramen magnum. When a patient's brain is injured, the resulting edema may cause it to swell, forcing brain tissue to herniate through either of these large foramina. Such a condition usually results in death.

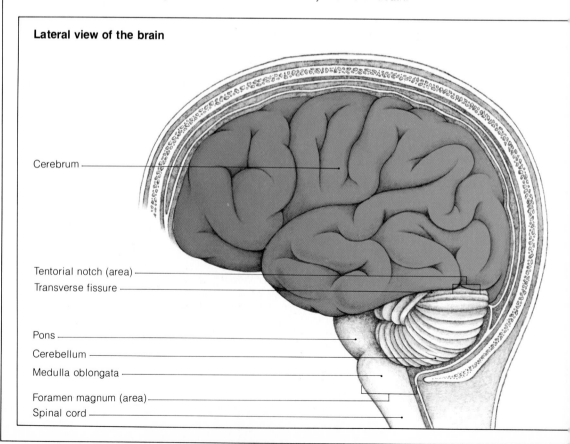

Lateral view of the brain

Cerebrum

Tentorial notch (area)

Transverse fissure

Pons

Cerebellum

Medulla oblongata

Foramen magnum (area)

Spinal cord

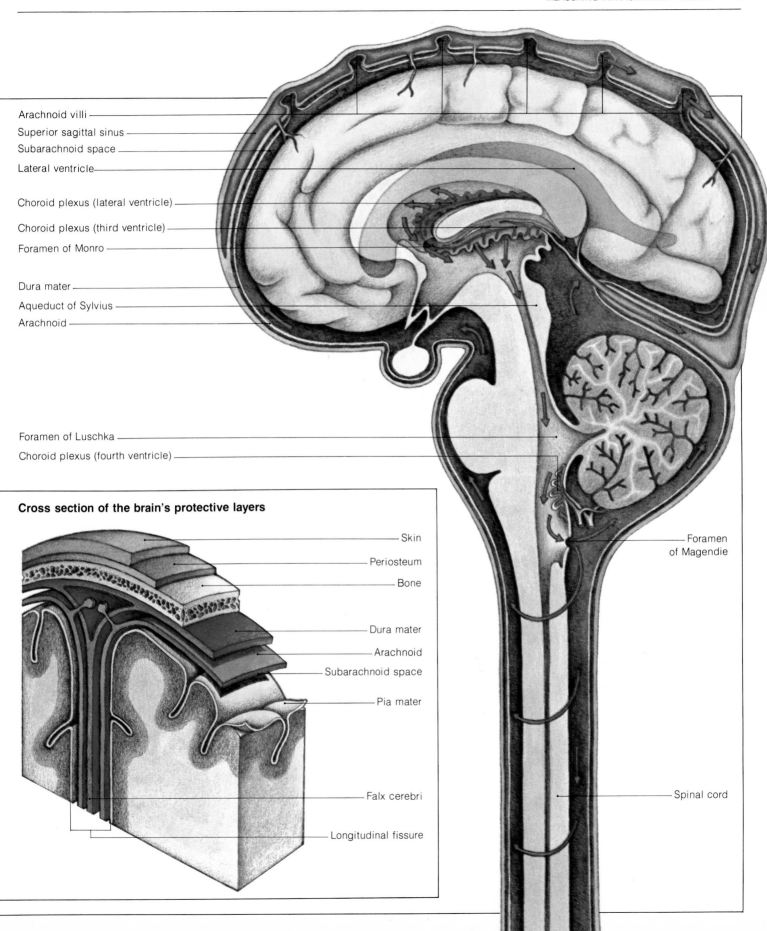

Arachnoid villi

Superior sagittal sinus

Subarachnoid space

Lateral ventricle

Choroid plexus (lateral ventricle)

Choroid plexus (third ventricle)

Foramen of Monro

Dura mater

Aqueduct of Sylvius

Arachnoid

Foramen of Luschka

Choroid plexus (fourth ventricle)

Foramen of Magendie

Spinal cord

Cross section of the brain's protective layers

Skin

Periosteum

Bone

Dura mater

Arachnoid

Subarachnoid space

Pia mater

Falx cerebri

Longitudinal fissure

Intracranial monitors

How the brain keeps intracranial pressure stable

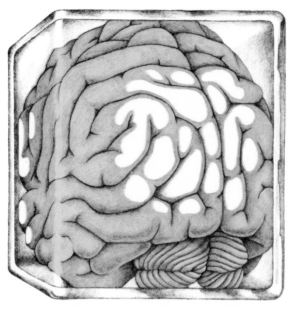

The brain is contained within the skull. Sound obvious? Certainly, but it's worth stressing, because it's one of the most important facts to remember about neurology. Think about it for a moment. The skull's an inflexible box. All its components—brain tissue, blood, and cerebrospinal fluid (CSF)—must coexist within very tight confines. A significant increase in the volume of any of these components must be offset by a decrease in one or both of the other components. If it's not, intracranial pressure (ICP) will rise quickly and dangerously.

What happens when a patient's ICP rises? The increased pressure prevents blood from perfusing the brain's cerebral cortex. As a result, the brain's deprived of its blood supply. For adequate perfusion, cerebral perfusion pressure (CPP) must be 60 to 90 mm Hg.

A patient undergoing ICP monitoring is probably undergoing continuous arterial blood pressure monitoring, too. You can calculate his CPP by subtracting ICP from his mean systemic arterial pressure (MSAP). Use this formula:

$$MSAP - ICP = CPP.$$

The brain accounts for about 85% of the skull's contents. Except in cases of disease or trauma, this proportion is fixed. So, ordinarily the brain compensates for increasing ICP by regulating the volume of blood and CSF with one of these mechanisms:

• *Pressure autoregulation.* Cerebral blood flow must remain stable, regardless of fluctuations in MSAP. If MSAP rises, the cerebral blood vessels constrict, limiting blood flow to the head. If necessary, the venous sinuses can collapse almost completely. Conversely, if MSAP falls, cerebral blood vessels dilate.

• *Metabolic autoregulation.* Receptors in the brain constantly analyze blood gases. If the level of wastes (CO_2 and lactic acid) rises, the cerebral blood vessels expand. As more blood reaches the brain, wastes are carried off and the oxygen level rises. Likewise, if the receptors detect a high level of oxygen in the blood, the cerebral blood vessels constrict and limit the flow of oxygen-carrying blood.

• *CSF regulation.* If ICP rises, CSF can be displaced into the spinal canal through several openings, primarily the foramen of Luschka and the foramen of Magendie. The dura that covers the spinal canal is loosely attached, and readily expands to accommodate departing CSF. At the same time, the arachnoid villi step up their absorption of CSF into the venous sinuses.

But what happens when the brain has reduced CSF and blood volume as much as possible? Then the brain begins to lose its ability to compensate for even small increases in volume. This inability to compensate is called decompensation, and a small increase in volume will produce a sharp, immediate rise in ICP.

Decompensation may also occur when ICP's too low; as a result, for example, of a sharp drop in MSAP. In such a case, pressure autoregulation may fail. Cerebral blood flow will then depend on MSAP, which has already fallen too low to maintain adequate CPP. Once again, the brain will be deprived of its blood supply.

Decompensation: A vicious cycle

During decompensation, the patient's cerebral blood flow is controlled by systemic arterial pressure (SAP) alone. So, if SAP rises (for any reason) during decompensation, the result may be a vicious, life-threatening cycle of rising intracranial pressure (ICP) and falling cerebral perfusion pressure (CPP). This illustration shows why.

• Responding to the rise in SAP, the patient's cerebral blood flow increases.

• This increase in blood flow increases his ICP.

• As his ICP rises, his CPP falls.

• Cerebral blood perfusion becomes inadequate, and the brain is deprived of its vital blood supply. As a result, the oxygen level in the brain drops, and CO_2 and lactic acid accumulate.

• Responding to this waste accumulation, the patient's cerebral blood vessels dilate, which further increases blood flow.

• The additional blood flow further increases ICP, and the cycle begins again.

How does the doctor evaluate decompensation? If the patient has a ventricular catheter in place, the doctor may perform a volume pressure response test. To do this, he'll first inject a small amount of sterile I.V. saline solution into the ventricular catheter. Then, he'll watch the monitor to see if the patient's ICP rises sharply in response to the sudden increase in intraventricular volume. If it does, the doctor will probably order immediate therapy to lower his patient's ICP. (To learn about different types of ICP therapy, study the chart on page 47.)

During decompensation, an increase in your patient's systemic arterial

pressure produces a dangerous spiral: His cerebral blood flow increases, his intracranial pressure increases,

his cerebral perfusion pressure decreases, his oxygen levels decrease, his carbon dioxide and lactic acid

levels increase (causing cerebral vasodilation), his cerebral blood flow increases, his intra-

cranial pressure increases, and his cerebral perfusion pressure decreases.

Intracranial monitors

Indications for ICP monitoring

As you know, your patient's brain, his cerebral blood supply, and his cerebrospinal fluid (CSF) are closely contained within his skull, an inflexible box. If he suffers from a condition that dramatically increases the volume of one or more of these components, his intracranial pressure (ICP) may rise to a dangerous level. In this case, he may need ICP monitoring.

Conditions that may require ICP monitoring include:
• massive brain lesion
• head trauma, with bleeding and edema
• congenital hydrocephalus
• encephalitis, especially Reye's syndrome
• cerebral hemorrhage
• overproduction and/or insufficient absorption of CSF, causing hydrocephalus.

ICP monitoring systems: Pros and cons

Are you familiar with the three most widely used intracranial pressure (ICP) monitoring systems? If not, this chart will acquaint you with their advantages and disadvantages.

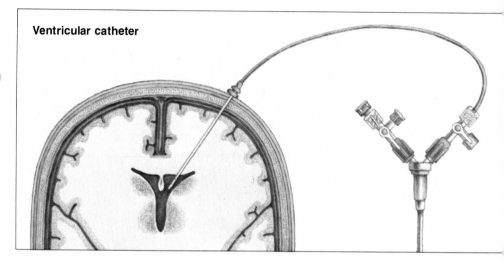

Ventricular catheter

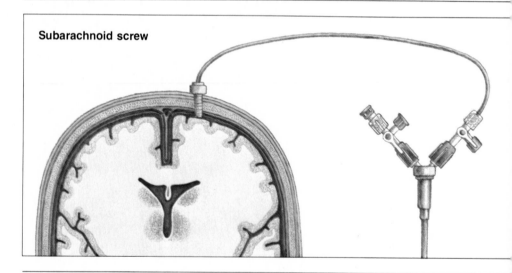

Subarachnoid screw

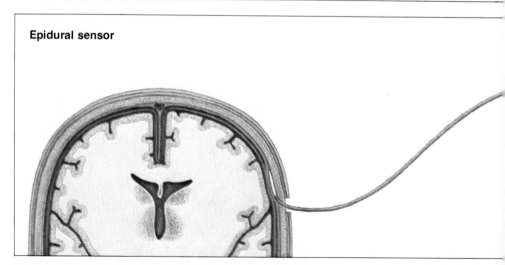

Epidural sensor

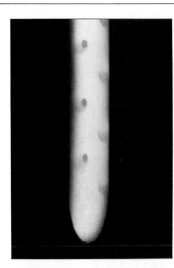

Advantages
* Measures ICP most accurately
* Evaluates volume/pressure responses
* Can drain large amounts of cerebrospinal fluid (CSF)
* Allows instillation of contrast media

Disadvantages
* Most invasive of the three monitoring systems; may expose patient to infections, such as ventriculitis or meningitis
* Catheter placement may be difficult, especially if the brain's ventricle is collapsed, swollen, or displaced.
* Drainage equipment provides an additional route for infection during treatment.
* Incorrect stopcock placement may allow excessive CSF drainage, causing a sudden drop in ICP. As a result, the brain may herniate.
* Catheter may become occluded with blood or brain tissue.
* Catheter may become compressed by the brain's collapsed ventricle, causing a false reading.
* Transducer and monitor must be recalibrated frequently.

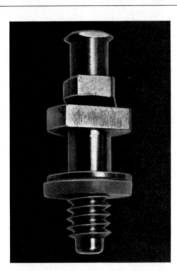

Advantages
* Measures ICP very accurately, directly from a CSF space
* Can be placed easily and quickly, without penetrating the cerebrum
* Provides access for CSF sampling

Disadvantages
* More invasive than epidural system, so it increases patient's risk of developing infection
* Can't drain significant amounts of CSF
* Can't evaluate volume/pressure responses reliably
* Screw may become occluded with blood or brain tissue.
* Transducer and monitor must be recalibrated frequently.

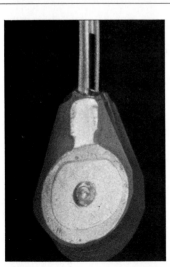

Advantages
* Easily placed in the epidural space
* Least invasive of the three systems, so it lessens patient's risk of developing infection
* Sensor can't become occluded with blood or CSF.
* Sensor and monitor don't require recalibration every time patient moves.

Disadvantages
* Reliability questionable. Although the sensor may be affected by heat or pressure, the system can't be recalibrated.
* Accuracy questionable. Doesn't measure pressure directly from a CSF space.
* Can't drain or sample CSF
* Can't evaluate volume/pressure responses
* Requires special equipment

Intracranial pressure setups: Some important reminders

Does one of your patients need intracranial pressure (ICP) monitoring? Chances are, the doctor will insert either a subarachnoid screw or a ventricular catheter. After that, he'll want you to set up the monitoring system.

As you know, inserting a screw or catheter is a surgical procedure. A catheter must be inserted in the OR, but a screw may be inserted in a critical care unit.

Setting up the monitoring system is your job. If you're unsure how, study the next two photostories carefully. But remember, these setting-up procedures may vary from hospital to hospital.

No matter what procedure you use, keep these important points in mind:
* Maintain sterile technique throughout. Do everything possible to reduce the risk of infection.
* Keep all stopcock ports capped, unless you must open one to expel air or balance the transducer. Before you begin setting up, replace any open stopcock caps with closed ones.
* Expel all air from the tubing and stopcock ports before connecting the line to the patient. Air in the line will damp the waveform, giving an inaccurate ICP reading.
* Never flush any fluid into the patient's cranial cavity. Doing so will raise his already elevated ICP and may invite infection, as well. (If the screw or catheter becomes occluded, notify the doctor. He may flush it with a small amount of sterile I.V. saline solution. Do not try to do this yourself.)

Note: Does your patient have an epidural sensor in place? Since this ICP measurement system isn't fluid-filled, you won't use either of the setting-up procedures explained in the next two photostories. To learn how to use an epidural sensor and to set up its monitoring system, turn to pages 40 and 41.

Intracranial monitors

How to set up equipment for subarachnoid ICP monitoring

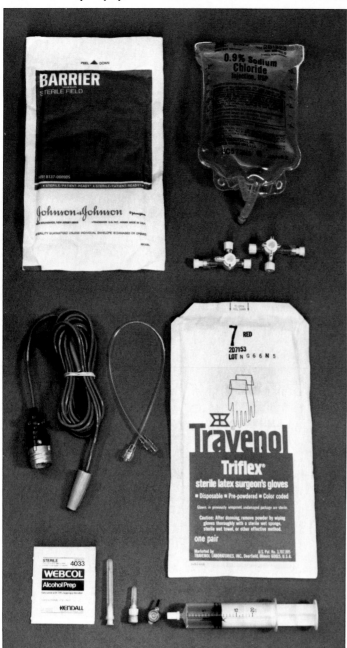

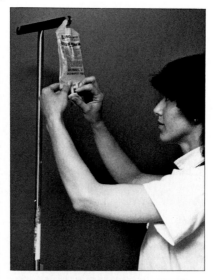

2 Spread the sterile towel over a table, to create a sterile field. Unwrap the equipment, and place it on the towel, observing sterile technique. *Remember:* Never contaminate a sterile field; for example, with unsterilized tape.

If the I.V. bag's in a sterile wrapper, unwrap it and place it on the sterile field. But if it's not sterile, like the one shown here, hang it on the I.V. pole. In either case, swab the injection port with the alcohol prep to prepare it for use.

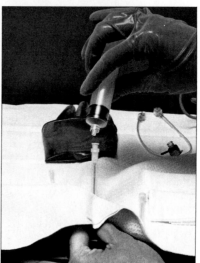

3 Now, slip a glove on your dominant hand. Place your ungloved hand under the sterile towel, and grasp the 18G needle, like the nurse is doing here. With your gloved hand, attach the 20 cc syringe to the needle, and remove the needle guard. Once again, place the needle guard on the sterile field.

1 *Whenever possible, ask another nurse to help you set up intracranial pressure (ICP) monitoring equipment. But when your unit's busy, you won't have that extra pair of hands. This photostory will show you how to meet the challenge alone.*

First, turn on the monitor, so it can warm up. (Like monitors, transducers need time to warm up. To save time, you may want to plug the transducer into the monitor now.)

Then, wash your hands thoroughly, and gather the equipment you see in this photo: a sterile towel, normal I.V. saline solution, two three-way stopcocks, a transducer, pressure tubing, sterile gloves, an 18G needle, an alcohol swab, a male adapter plug, a minidome, and a 20 cc syringe. In addition, you'll need an I.V. pole.

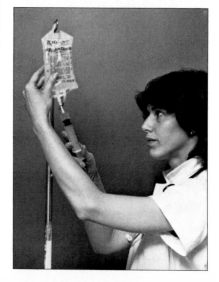

4 Next, steady the I.V. bag with your ungloved hand. Remember, the bag's not sterile, so don't touch it with your sterile glove. Using your gloved hand, insert the needle into the bag's injection port, and withdraw 20 ml saline solution.

5 Then, carefully scoop up the needle guard with the needle, and attach it securely. Remove the needle from the syringe and discard it (away from the sterile field). *Important:* As you work, take care not to contaminate the syringe with your ungloved hand.

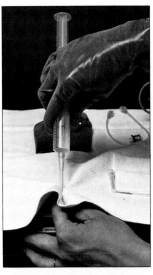

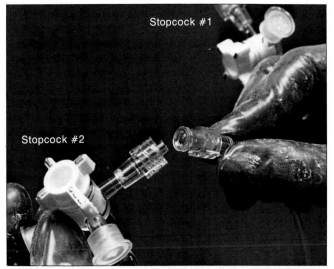

8 Attach the Luer-Lok™ port of the second stopcock to the other end of the pressure tubing. For clarity, we'll call the stopcock closer (proximal) to the patient *Stopcock #1,* and the one closer to the monitor (distal to the patient) *Stopcock #2,* as labeled in this photo.

6 Place the syringe on the sterile field. Then, slip a glove on your other hand.

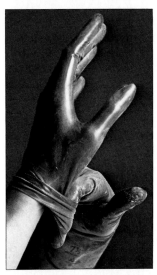

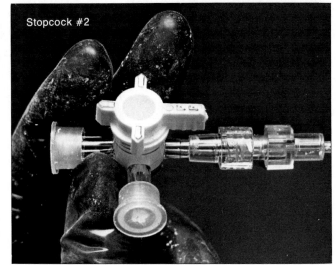

9 Turn the handles on Stopcock #2 closed to the pressure tubing, as shown here. Now the line's open between the middle and lateral ports of Stopcock #2 and closed to the pressure tubing.

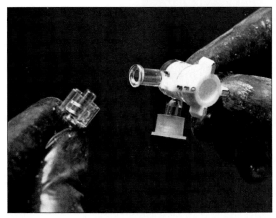

7 Attach the pressure tubing to the lateral port of one of the stopcocks, as shown here. (Remember, tighten all connections securely to minimize the risk of disconnection.)

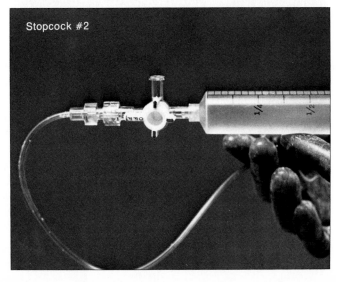

10 Attach the 20 cc syringe to the lateral port of Stopcock #2, as the nurse has done here. Then, take the cap off the middle port.

Intracranial monitors

How to set up equipment for subarachnoid ICP monitoring continued

11 Holding the middle port of Stopcock #2 upright, depress the syringe plunger and flush the middle port with saline solution. (The upright position of the port encourages air bubbles to rise and escape.)

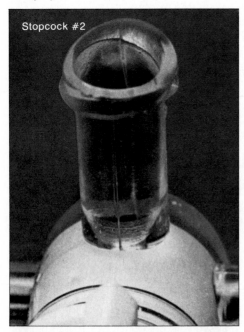

Stopcock #2

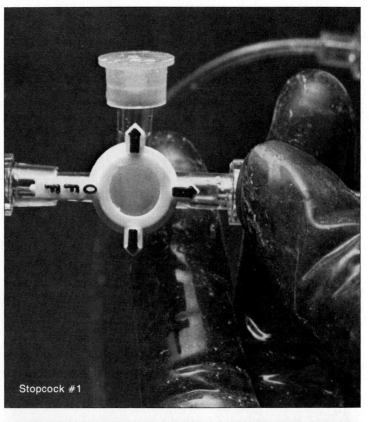

Stopcock #1

13 Turn the handle of Stopcock #1 off to its Luer-Lok port. Now, the line's open between the lateral port of Stopcock #2 and the middle port of Stopcock #1. Uncap the middle port of Stopcock #1.

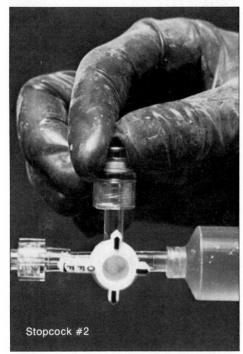

Stopcock #2

12 When all the air's been expelled from the middle port, cap it with the disposable minidome. Then, turn the handle off to the middle port.

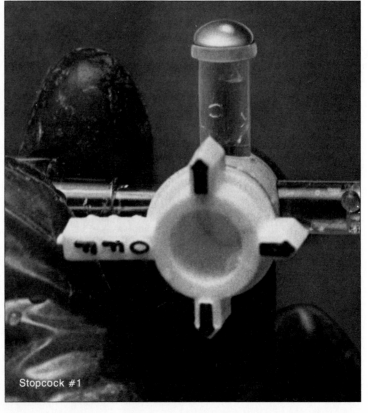

Stopcock #1

14 Using the syringe, flush the middle port of Stopcock #1 with saline solution, remembering to hold the port upright, so air can escape easily. Tap out all air bubbles, and look for a meniscus.

15 Turn the handle of Stopcock #1 off to the middle port. Then attach the male adapter plug (nipple port) to the middle port.

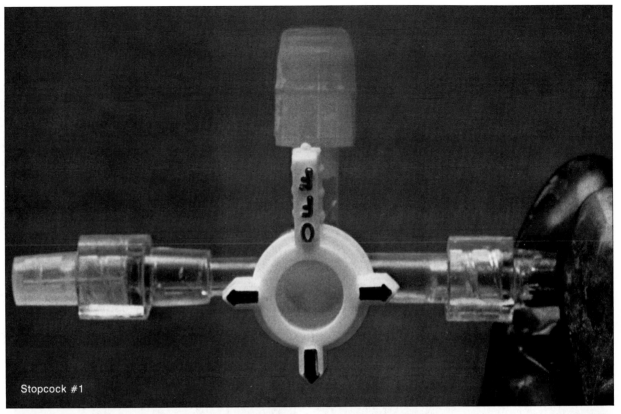

Stopcock #1

16 Hold the Luer-Lok port of Stopcock #1 upright, and flush it with saline solution.

Cap the Luer-Lok port.

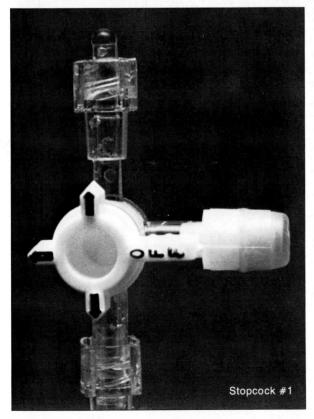

Stopcock #1

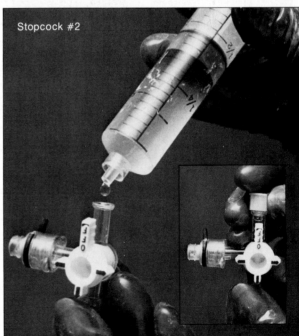

Stopcock #2

17 Turn Stopcock #2 off to the syringe, and remove the syringe. To expel air from this port, drop sterile saline solution in it, as the nurse is doing here.

[Inset] When it's completely filled with saline solution and you see a meniscus, cap the port.

Intracranial monitors

How to set up equipment for subarachnoid ICP monitoring continued

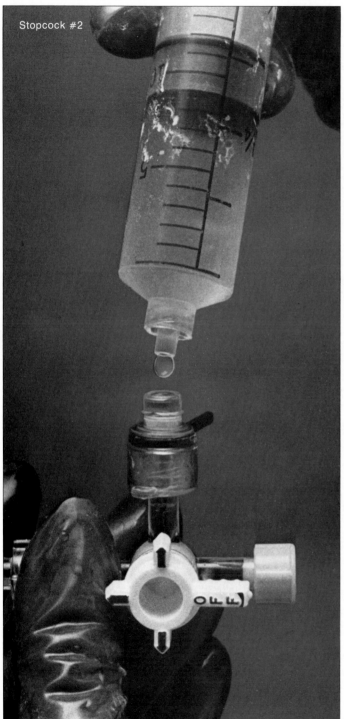

18 Now, you're ready to attach the transducer to the mini-dome on Stopcock #2. Using the syringe, drop sterile saline solution into the minidome's cylinder, until a meniscus forms. *Note:* If you're using a standard-sized transducer dome, completely fill it—as well as both its arms—with saline solution. Remember, air bubbles must be expelled from every portion of the system.

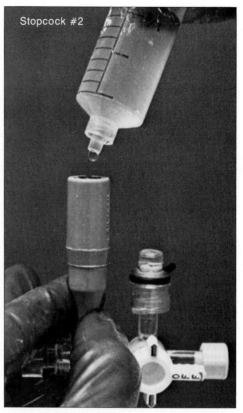

19 Continue to hold the mini-dome upright. At the same time, fill the inside of the transducer with saline solution, until a meniscus forms. (Filling both the mini-dome and the transducer with saline solution reduces the chance of trapping air during connection.)

If you're using a standard-sized transducer and dome, do not fill the transducer itself with saline solution. Instead, place several drops of the solution on the transducer diaphragm—but not too much, or the saline solution will distort the waveform.

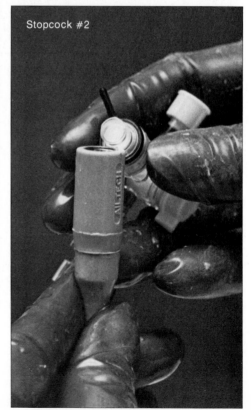

20 Hold the transducer upright. As you continue to do so, screw the mini-dome into the transducer.

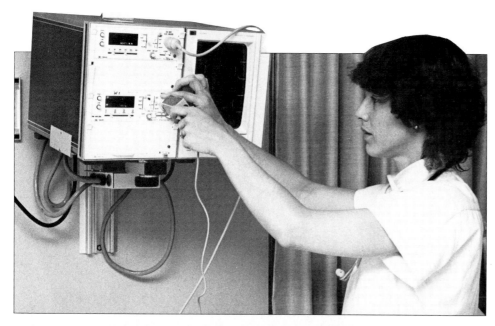

21 Now, plug in the transducer, if you haven't done so already. The doctor will fill the Luer-Lok port of Stopcock #1 with saline solution and connect it tightly to the subarachnoid screw—or to the extension tubing attached to the screw. *Important:* After the system's connected to your patient, watch stopcock positioning carefully. *Never* allow fluid to enter your patient's cranial cavity.

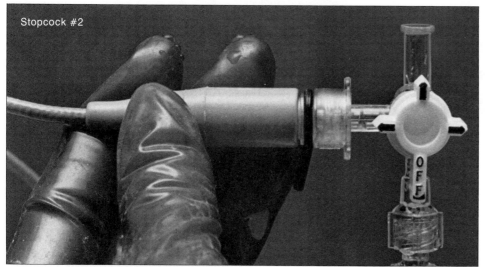

Stopcock #2

22 To balance the transducer, turn Stopcock #2 so it's open between the lateral port and the transducer, and closed to Stopcock #1. Place Stopcock #2 so its lateral port is upright and level with the patient's foramen of Monro (between the edge of the eyebrow and the ear's tragus). Uncap the lateral port of Stopcock #2, as shown here. Balance the transducer and cap the lateral port of Stopcock #2. Calibrate the transducer with the monitor.

Important: Always position the balancing port (in this case, the lateral port of Stopcock #2)—not the transducer itself—level with the foramen of Monro.

Secure the stopcocks and transducer at the same level you used for balancing. Remember, if the patient's position changes, reposition and rebalance the transducer and recalibrate it with the monitor.

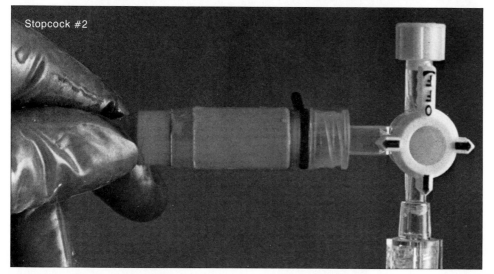

Stopcock #2

23 Now you're ready to monitor your patient's ICP. Turn both stopcock handles so the line's open between the patient and the monitor. This photo shows the handle position for Stopcock #2.

Who applies the dressing to the insertion site? The doctor will probably apply it himself. But if he wants you to do it, follow the procedure shown on page 38.

Thoroughly document the entire procedure in your nurses' notes. To reduce the risk of infection, change the setup and dressing once daily for as long as the subarachnoid screw is in place. The doctor will probably remove the screw (or replace it) within 5 days.

Intracranial monitors

Setting up equipment for ventricular ICP monitoring

1 *If your patient has a ventricular catheter in place, the doctor will want you to connect a drainage bag to the line. This way, he can drain excess cerebrospinal fluid (CSF), as well as monitor intracranial pressure (ICP). In this photostory, you'll see how to set up a line that'll accommodate a monitor and a drainage bag.*

To begin, turn on the monitor and plug in the transducer, so they can warm up. Then, wash your hands and gather the equipment listed below. Establish a sterile field, and place all sterile equipment on it. Remember to maintain sterile technique throughout the procedure.

Drainage bag (emptied 500 ml bag of sterile I.V. saline solution, without injection port)

500 ml bag of normal saline solution

Two three-way stopcocks

Minidome

Minitransducer

Sterile towel

Macrodrip I.V. tubing

1'' pressure tubing

Extra stopcock port caps

Sterile gloves

20 cc syringe

Sterile 18G needle

Alcohol prep

2'' wide tape (optional)

Povidone-iodine prep (optional)

Sterile 4'' x 4'' gauze pads (optional)

Male adapter plug (optional)

4'' roller gauze (optional)

2 Now, slip a glove on one hand. Use the syringe to withdraw 20 ml sterile I.V. saline solution, using the technique shown on pages 26 and 27. Slip a glove on the other hand, and connect the two stopcocks to each other. Then, connect the pressure tubing to one of the stopcocks. Later, the doctor will connect the pressure tubing to the patient's catheter.

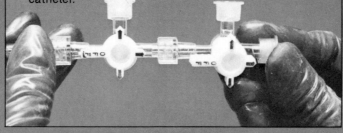

3 Get ready to flush the stopcocks. (For easy reference, we'll call the stopcock closer [proximal] to the patient *Stopcock #1;* and the distal one *Stopcock #2*, as labeled in this photo.)

Turn the stopcock handles so the line's open between the lateral port of Stopcock #2 and the middle port of Stopcock #1. Use the syringe to expel the air from the middle port of Stopcock #1.

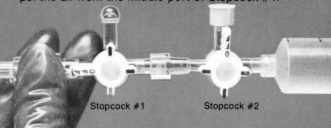

Stopcock #1   Stopcock #2

4 Cap the middle stopcock port on Stopcock #1 with the minidome.

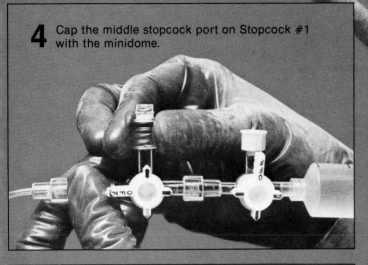

6 Use the syringe to expel all the air from the pressure tubing. Cap the tubing (see inset).

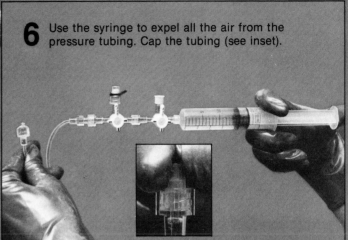

5 Turn Stopcock #1 off to the dome. Now, the line's open to the pressure tubing.

Stopcock #1   Stopcock #2

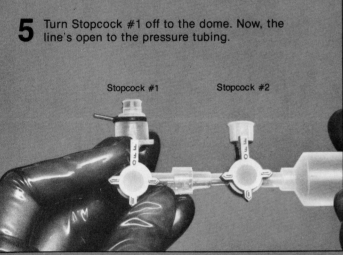

7 Turn Stopcock #2 off to Stopcock #1, as shown here. Use the syringe to expel air from the middle port of Stopcock #2; then cap the port. *Note:* If the doctor wants an injection port on the line, cap the middle port of Stopcock #2 with a male adapter plug (nipple port).

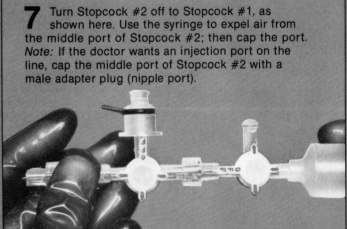

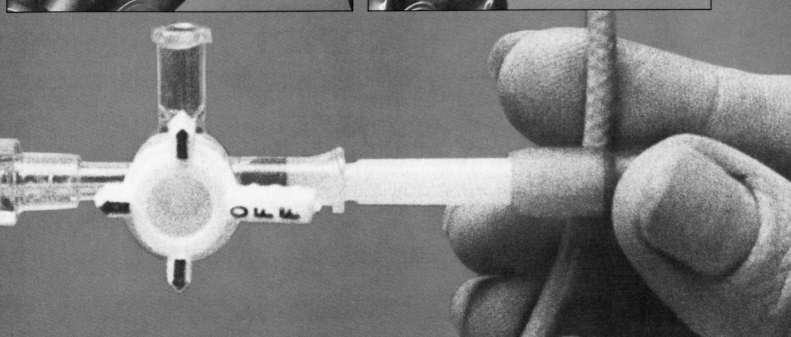

Intracranial monitors

Setting up equipment for ventricular ICP monitoring continued

8 Next, turn Stopcock #2 off to the middle port, and remove the syringe. Drop saline solution from the syringe into the lateral port, until it's full of saline solution and free of air. Then, cap the port (see inset). Now both stopcocks and the pressure tubing are completely flushed.

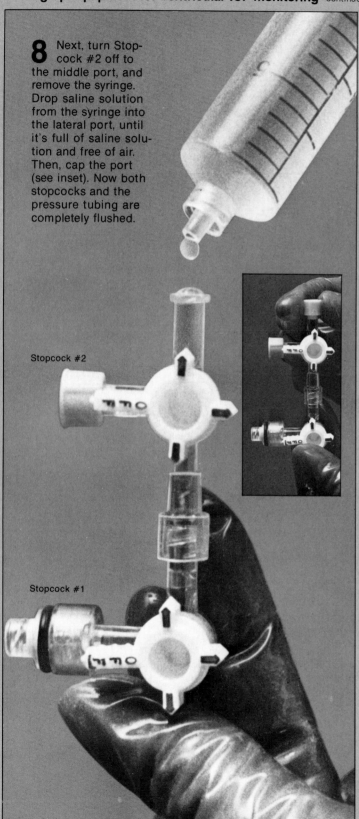

Stopcock #2

Stopcock #1

9 Use the syringe to fill the top of the dome with saline solution, forming a meniscus. Fill the transducer with saline solution, and form a meniscus in it too (see inset).

Stopcock #1

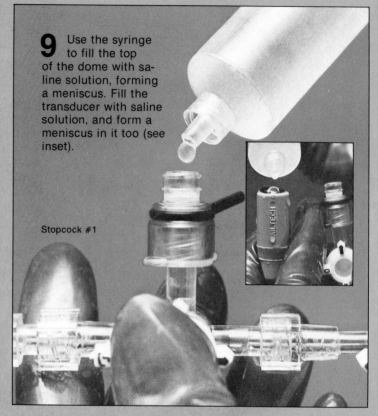

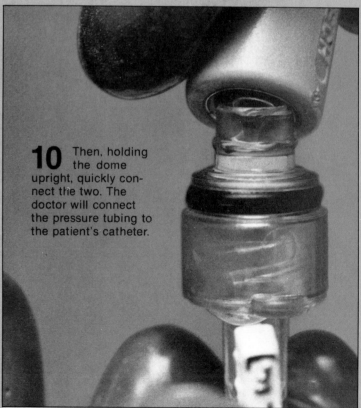

10 Then, holding the dome upright, quickly connect the two. The doctor will connect the pressure tubing to the patient's catheter.

11 Now you're ready to attach the drainage bag. Make sure the clamp on the macrodrip I.V. tubing's closed; then spike the drainage bag. Attach the other end of the I.V. tubing to the lateral port of Stopcock #2. Putting the drainage bag on the stopcock port most distal to the patient facilitates drainage by providing a straight pathway through the stopcocks. Now the bag's ready to receive CSF drainage, if the doctor orders.

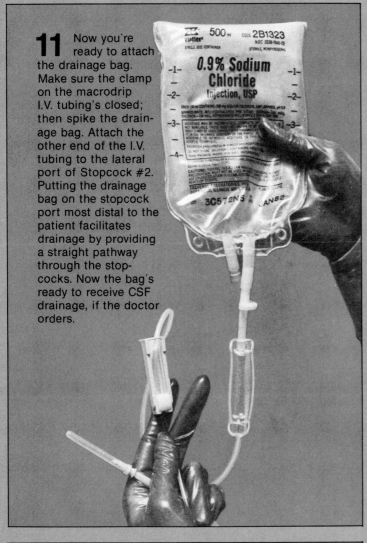

12 Open the line between the middle port of Stopcock #2 and the transducer, and close the line to the patient. Place the middle port of Stopcock #2 level with the patient's foramen of Monro. Next, open this port to air and balance the transducer. (Since this is not a sterile procedure, you can remove your gloves, as the nurse has done here.)

Stopcock #1   Stopcock #2

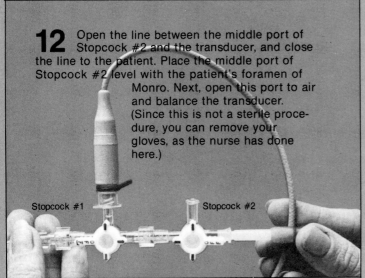

13 Cap Stopcock #2's middle port, and calibrate the transducer with the monitor. (Since the monitor's buttons aren't sterile, always do this step last.) Then, open the line between the patient and the transducer, and begin ICP monitoring. Document the procedure thoroughly in your nurses' notes.

Important: To guard against infection, change all equipment and the patient's dressing daily. (To learn how to change a dressing, see page 38.) In addition, send a properly labeled CSF sample to the lab every day for culturing. To learn how to drain CSF, read the next photostory.

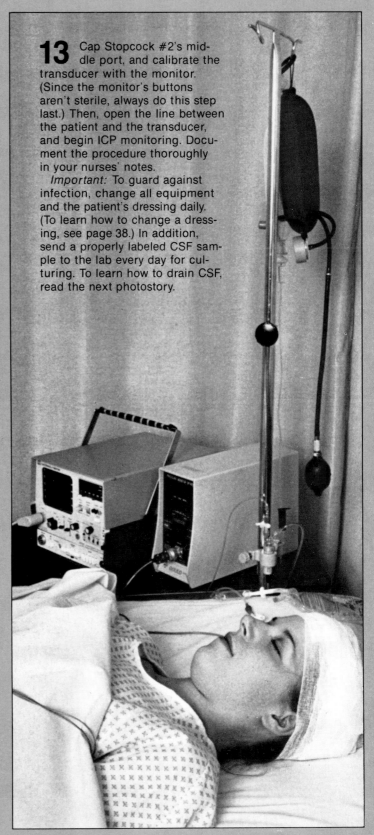

Intracranial monitors

Draining cerebrospinal fluid (CSF) through a ventricular catheter

1 *As you know, you can use a ventricular catheter to drain CSF, as well as for intracranial pressure (ICP) monitoring. In the preceding photostory, you learned how to assemble the equipment. Here's how to use it:*
    First, locate the stopcock farther from the patient (Stopcock #2). Then, make sure the handle on this stopcock reads OFF to the middle port.

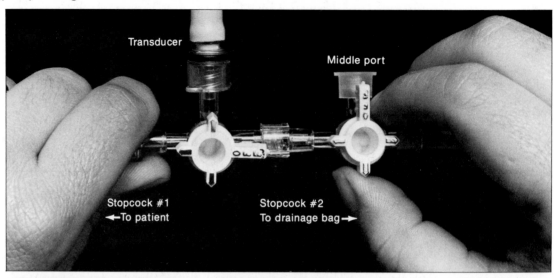

2 Turn the handle of Stopcock #1 OFF to the transducer. Now, the line's open between your patient and the drainage bag.

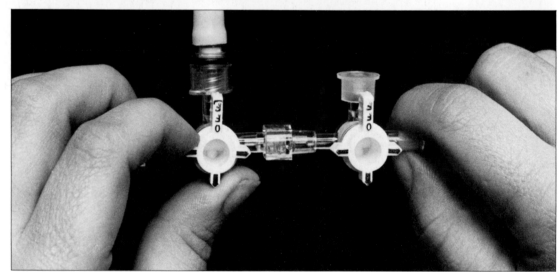

3 Open the clamp on the drainage bag tubing, and allow the CSF to drain.
    Important: Monitor CSF drainage closely. Excessive drainage produces a false low ICP reading. Under certain conditions, excessive drainage may also cause brain herniation.

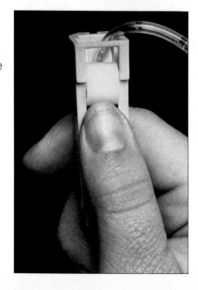
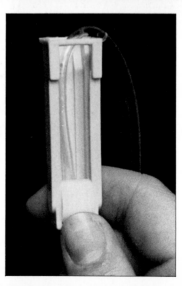

4 When you've drained CSF according to the doctor's orders, close the clamp on the drainage tubing.

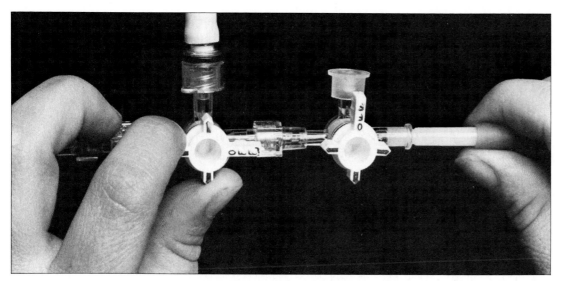

5 Turn the handle of Stopcock #1 OFF to the drainage bag. Leave the handle of Stopcock #2 as it is. Now, the line between the patient and the transducer is open again, and you can resume monitoring.

6 Document the procedure, including the amount of CSF drained. Send the properly labeled CSF sample to the lab for culturing. (Do this at least once every 24 hours.)
Important: Never open the drainage bag to obtain a sample. This risks infection. Instead, remove the bag entirely from the setup, and replace it with a new sterile bag.

Patient's name: **Alice Decker**   Age: **61**

Room #: **334**   Doctor: **R. Brownstein**

Date	Time	Nurses' Notes
6-18-80	4PM	ICP increased to 40 mm Hg and sustained for 20 minutes. Decerebrate response to pain. Bradycardia at 54 beats per min. B/P 184/100. Dr. Brownstein notified. Ordered existing ventriculostomy opened to drain CSF until ICP returns to normal.
	5PM	ICP down to 36 mm Hg. CSF clear. Heart rate 70 beats/min.; B/P 174/94. Patient moves extremities randomly. Decerebrate response to pain.
	6PM	ICP down to 12 mm Hg for past 5 minutes. Heart rate 74 beats/min.; B/P 160/90. Decerebrate response to pain continues. Total of 30 ml CSF drained. Dr. Brownstein notified of ICP reading and amount of CSF drained. Dr. ordered CSF to be sent to Lab for culture and sensitivity tests. Drainage bag removed and new drainage bag applied to patient's line. (CSF specimen sent to Lab.) M. Klevence, RN

Intracranial monitors

How to apply a head bandage

1 *Most likely, the doctor will put a head bandage on your patient after he completes the surgical procedure necessary for ICP catheter or screw insertion. But he'll expect you to change the dressing daily, if it's a nursing responsibility in your hospital. Remember to maintain sterile technique throughout. Here's what to do:*

Gather the equipment shown in this photo. Open all the sterile wrappers, and lay the items on the bedside table so the *inside* of the wrappers face up. This way, each piece of equipment has its own sterile field. *Remember:* Don't touch any sterile equipment (including the inside of the wrappers) with your hands.

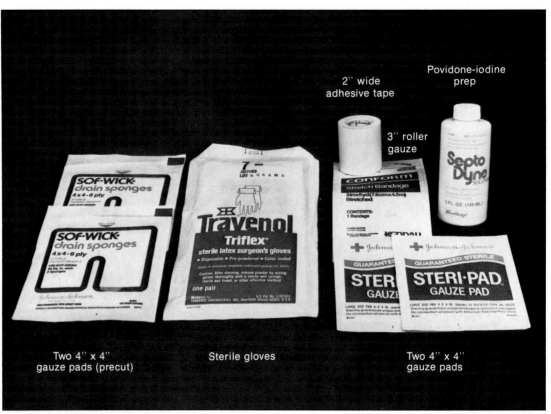

2" wide
adhesive tape

Povidone-iodine
prep

3" roller
gauze

Two 4" x 4"
gauze pads (precut)

Sterile gloves

Two 4" x 4"
gauze pads

2 Without touching the uncut gauze pads, saturate them with povidone-iodine, as shown in the inset. Then, remove the patient's old dressing and dispose of it properly.

Slip gloves on your hands. Then, pick up the saturated pads and dab povidone-iodine around the catheter's or screw's insertion site, as the nurse is doing in the large illustration. As you work, examine the site carefully for any signs of infection, swelling, irritation, or drainage. If you see anything unusual, tell the doctor at once.

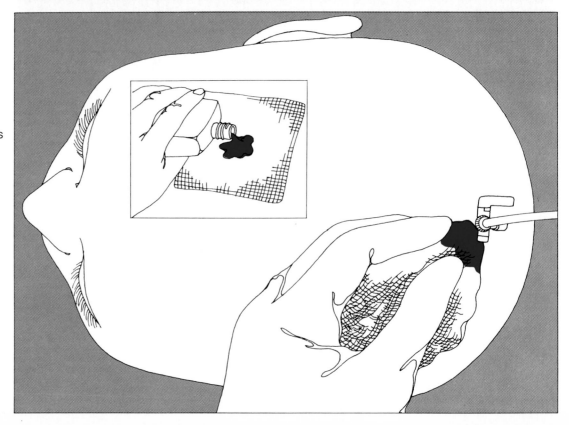

3 Now, place the two precut gauze pads around the screw or catheter (as shown here), so their edges completely overlap.

Make sure the screw or catheter is fully exposed and easily accessible.

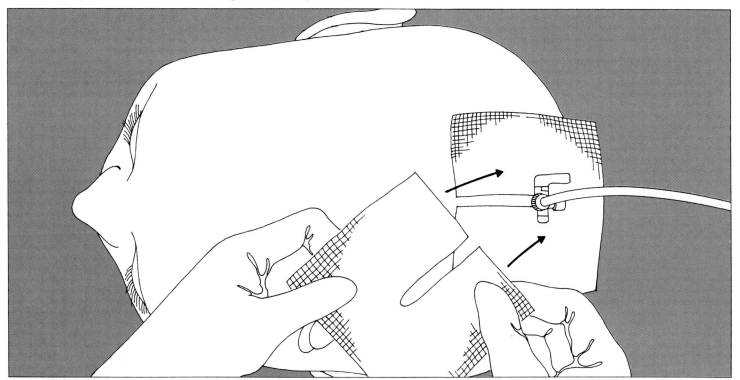

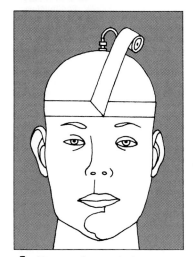

4 Now you're ready to secure the gauze pads with roller gauze. Starting at the back of your patient's head, wrap the roller gauze around his head twice. Stop rolling the gauze when it's in the center of his forehead.

Then, fold the gauze so it's pointing up, and begin rolling it across the patient's crown, as shown here.

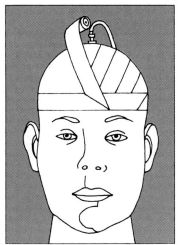

5 When you reach the back of your patient's head, hold the gauze down with one finger, and reverse the procedure, bringing the gauze to the front of your patient's head. Repeat this process several times until one side of your patient's head is covered by the gauze. Double the gauze back across the forehead to the other side.

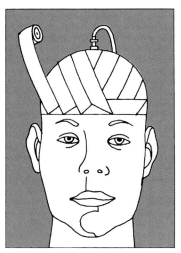

6 Then, repeat the wrapping process on the other side of your patient's head. *Remember:* Leave the catheter or screw exposed.

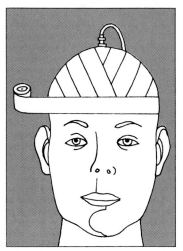

7 Now, wrap the roller gauze around your patient's head again, to secure the folded corners. Secure the end of the roller gauze with a single piece of tape. Document the dressing change in your nurses' notes.

Intracranial monitors

Learning about an epidural monitoring system

The epidural intracranial pressure (ICP) monitoring system shown in the next photostory is manufactured by Ladd Research Industries, Inc. It has two essential parts: an epidural fiberoptic sensor and a monitor. The monitor may be connected to a pen recorder (Houston Instrument Co.) to produce pressure readout strips.

The doctor implants the tiny fiberoptic sensor in the epidural space, through a small burr hole in the patient's skull. To avoid wedging (compressing) the sensor, the doctor carefully strips, or separates, the brain's dura layers. When he's finished, you can plug the sensor cable directly into the monitor.

How does this particular monitoring system work? Look at the illustration of the sensor below. Light from the monitor is transmitted to the sensor through fibers in the cable. A mirror on the sensor's internal diaphragm reflects the light, which travels back to the monitor through the fibers in the cable. Since the mirror changes position in response to the patient's ICP, the intensity of the reflected light varies. A transducer in the monitor analyzes these variations, after which the monitor converts them into a continuous numerical display.

Fiberoptic sensors of this type may be sterilized and reused several times. However, check their accuracy before each use. To do this, set the monitor on MANUAL TEST and apply a known pressure to the sensor with a fluid reservoir; then, compare the monitor reading to the known pressure. If the readings aren't identical, discard the sensor; the system can't be recalibrated.

In the following photostory, you'll learn how to use this ICP monitoring system. Once you use this system, you'll discover it has lots of advantages. Besides being easy to assemble and operate, it's far less invasive than either the screw or the catheter. And because the system has no fluid path or electrical wiring between the patient and the monitor, it presents no electrical hazard. Although relatively new, the Ladd epidural ICP monitoring system has been used successfully at many hospitals.

Nevertheless, epidural ICP monitoring remains controversial. In the past, this type of ICP monitoring system was plagued with serious drift problems that could not be remedied, since the system can't be recalibrated. Today, the new epidural ICP monitoring systems have been improved. But since the fiberoptic sensor doesn't contact a CSF space, some doctors still doubt the system's ability to measure ICP accurately.

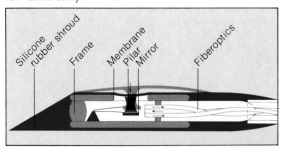

How to use an epidural monitoring system

If the doctor implants a fiberoptic epidural sensor, he'll expect you to connect the sensor's cable to the monitor and begin monitoring. Do you know how? Just follow these steps:

Before you begin, take a look at the monitor's front panel. Make sure the POWER switch is off and the AUTO SENSOR switch is on, as shown below. (Notice the small numbers set inside triangular designs at the upper right corner and along the monitor's base. Follow them to identify the steps needed to set up the system. Also, use them as a guide for following this photostory (the first step's to your *right*).

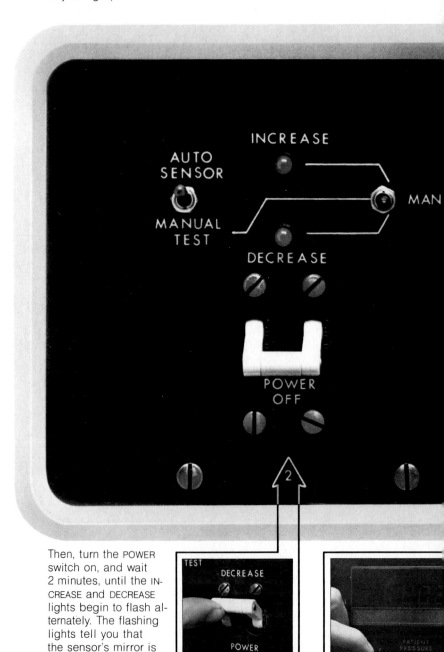

Then, turn the POWER switch on, and wait 2 minutes, until the INCREASE and DECREASE lights begin to flash alternately. The flashing lights tell you that the sensor's mirror is changing position in response to intracranial pressure (ICP).

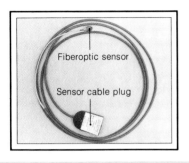

Fiberoptic sensor

Sensor cable plug

In the upper right corner (beneath the number 1), you'll see the cable receptacle for the plug on the sensor's cable. Hold the plug so the label faces up, and insert the plug into the cable receptacle, as shown on the right.

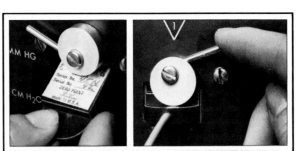

Turn the cable receptacle's latch to the right, until it locks. With the cable locked in place, the monitoring system's now connected to the patient.

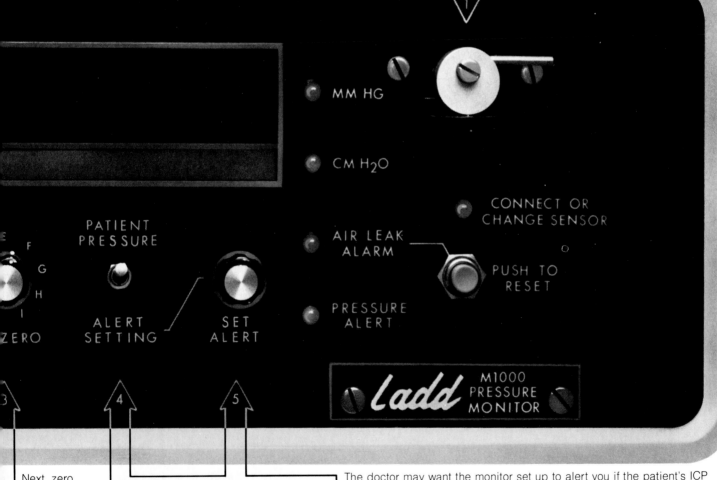

Next, zero the epidural sensor by adjusting the SET ZERO knob until the digital reading is between −1 and +2.

The doctor may want the monitor set up to alert you if the patient's ICP reaches a predetermined level. If so, here's what to do. Hold down the PATIENT PRESSURE switch with one hand. With your other hand, turn the SET ALERT knob until the pressure level the doctor's indicated appears on the digital reading. Then, release the PATIENT PRESSURE switch.

When you release the PATIENT PRESSURE switch, the monitor will automatically display the patient's ICP. But if his ICP reaches the pressure level set on the monitor, the PRESSURE ALERT light will flash. (You can change this pressure level at any time by repeating this procedure.)

Finally, document the procedure in your nurses' notes.

Intracranial monitors

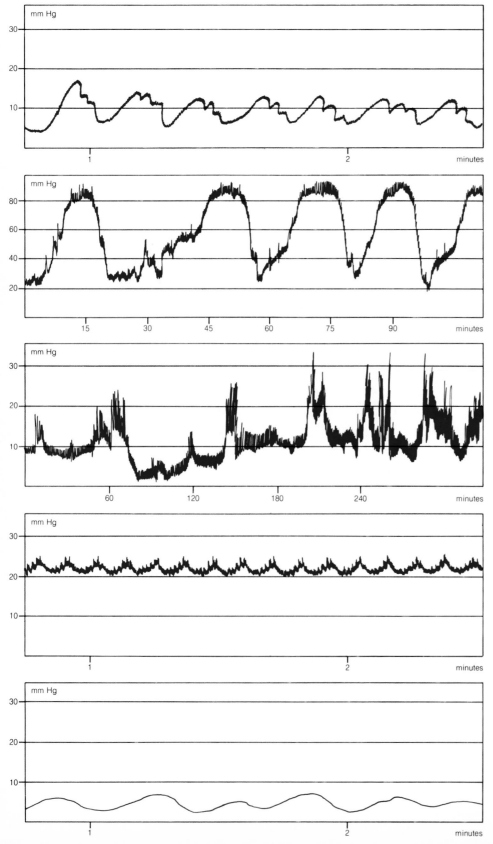

Reading ICP waveforms accurately

1 *When you monitor a patient's intracranial pressure (ICP), you'll see some or all of the waveforms illustrated here.* Pictured to the left is a normal ICP waveform. Notice the steep upward systolic slope, followed by the downward diastolic slope with dicrotic notch. Ordinarily, this waveform occurs continuously and indicates an ICP measurement between 4 and 15 mm Hg.

2 The A waves shown here (sometimes called plateau waves) typically reach elevations of 50 to 100 mm Hg; and then drop sharply. They may come and go as the result of a temporary rise in thoracic pressure. But if they're recurring or are sustained for several minutes, A waves indicate a rapid, dangerous rise in ICP and a decreased ability to compensate. Consider such waves ominous. Notify the doctor at once. Sustained A waves may indicate irreversible brain damage.

3 The B waves illustrated here are sharp and rhythmic, with a sawtooth pattern. They occur every 1½ to 2 minutes and may reach elevations of 50 mm Hg. However, these high elevations aren't sustained. The clinical significance of B waves isn't clear, but they seem to occur more frequently with decreasing compensation. Sometimes, they precede A waves. Watch them closely, so you can notify the doctor promptly if such a change occurs.

4 C waves, as shown here, are rapid and rhythmic. They're less sharp in appearance than B waves, and may fluctuate with respirations or changing systemic blood pressure. C waves aren't clinically significant.

5 This illustration shows a damped waveform. This waveform tells you that the line's obstructed or that the transducer needs rebalancing. Locate the problem, and try to correct it. (For troubleshooting tips on how to do this, see the chart on page 44.)

ICP readings: What's normal?

As you know, the normal range for intracranial pressure (ICP) readings is between 4 and 15 mm Hg (5 to 20 cm H_2O). But that's variable. ICP readings can fluctuate as much as 20 mm Hg, even in healthy people. And many everyday activities—for example, isometric exercises, straining at bowel movements, even sustained coughing—can temporarily spike ICP readings even higher.

When you monitor a patient with high ICP readings, remember that the *pattern* of readings is more significant than any *single* reading. By comparing a series of ICP readings, determine what's normal for your patient. Then, if you observe *elevated* ICP readings, pay particular attention to how long they're sustained. If they're sustained for several minutes, notify the doctor immediately so he can begin treatment.

DOCUMENTING

Documenting ICP measurements

Depending on your hospital's equipment and policy, you may document intracranial pressure (ICP) measurements in your nurses' notes, on a flow chart, or directly on readout strips. The following is a sample of proper documentation, using a flow chart and a readout strip.

Using a flow chart. If your patient's undergoing ICP monitoring, he's probably also undergoing hemodynamic monitoring—and of course, routine urine output and vital signs monitoring, as well. Documenting his care on a flow chart, like the one shown below, lets you assess his progress (or lack of it) at a glance. As you can see, space exists at the bottom of the chart to document anything that may affect pressure readings, vital signs, or urine output; for example, drug therapy, stressful nursing procedures, or sleep.

Patient: *Arthur Parrish*   Room number: *365*

Time	Temperature, pulse, and respiration (TPR)	Blood pressure (B/P)	Central venous pressure (CVP)	Mean pulmonary artery pressure (MPAP)	Pulmonary artery wedge pressure (PAWP)	Intracranial pressure (ICP)	Urine output
10 PM	99-104-22	150/90	10.5 mm Hg	16 mm Hg	7.5 mm Hg	9 mm Hg	51 ml
11 PM	92-24	180/90	12.5 mm Hg	18 mm Hg	10 mm Hg	40 mm Hg	33 ml
11:30 PM	86-20	154/92	10.5 mm Hg	17 mm Hg	8 mm Hg	10 mm Hg	39 ml
12 MIDNIGHT	103-90-32	180/94	10.5 mm Hg	18 mm Hg	8.5 mm Hg	8 mm Hg	42 ml
1 AM	142-40	212/102	13 mm Hg	20 mm Hg	12 mm Hg	72 mm Hg	22 ml
1:30 AM	100-26	160/92	11 mm Hg	17 mm Hg	9 mm Hg	12 mm Hg	38 ml

11 PM - Patient suctioned and turned. ICP increased to 40 mm Hg for 5 minutes, then returned to 10 mm Hg.
1 AM - Patient fighting ET tube and coughing. Suctioned and bagged patient using 100% O_2. Patient ICP increased to 72 mm Hg for 7 minutes postepisode. ICP then decreased to 12 mm Hg, and patient rested quietly.

Using a readout strip. If the monitor's connected to a recorder, document patient care on the readout strip too. This'll help you determine how well the patient responds to therapy and how he reacts to day-to-day procedures.

For example, suppose the doctor administers mannitol to decrease the patient's ICP. Note the exact time the doctor administers the mannitol on the readout strip, as shown on this sample. Then you'll have an accurate, handy record of how well—and how quickly—the patient responded to therapy.

In addition, document periods of coughing, suctioning, and combativeness, as well as any nursing procedure that may spike your patient's ICP. That way, you have a record of how these stresses affect your patient's ICP.

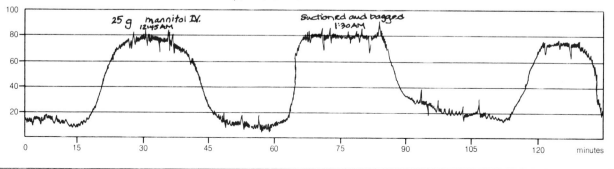

Intracranial monitors

How to troubleshoot a damped waveform

Possible cause	Solution
Transducer or monitor needs recalibration	• Turn stopcock off to patient. • Open transducer's stopcock to air, and balance transducer. • Recalibrate transducer and monitor.
Air in line	• Turn stopcock off to patient. • Using a syringe, flush air out through an open stopcock port with sterile I.V. saline solution. *Note:* Never use heparin to flush the ICP line. You could accidentally inject some of the drug into the patient and cause bleeding. • Rebalance and recalibrate transducer and monitor.
Loose connection in line	• Check tubing and stopcocks for possible moisture, which may indicate a loose connection. • Turn stopcock off to patient; then tighten all connections. • Make sure the tubing's long enough to allow patient to turn his head without straining the tubing. This may prevent further problems.
Disconnection in line	• Turn stopcock off to patient *immediately*. (Rapid CSF loss through a ventricular catheter may allow ICP to drop precipitously, causing brain herniation.) • Replace equipment to reduce risk of infection.
Change in patient's position	• Reposition transducer's balancing port level with foramen of Monro. • Rebalance and recalibrate transducer and monitor. *Remember:* Always balance and recalibrate at least once every 4 hours, and whenever the patient's repositioned.
Tubing, catheter, or screw occluded with blood or brain tissue	• Notify doctor. He may want to irrigate the screw or catheter with a small amount (0.1 ml) of sterile I.V. saline solution. *Important:* Never irrigate the screw or catheter yourself.

Assessing your patient's progress

In most cases, intracranial pressure (ICP) monitoring signals the first warning of rising ICP. That's why you can't assume your patient's OK just because he doesn't show clinical signs of distress.

But that doesn't mean clinical signs are unimportant. Your skill at assessing changes in the patient's condition is essential for complete care. As always, *watch the patient as closely as you watch his monitor.*

The first sign of rising ICP may be headache or vomiting. But consider *any* changes in the patient's general condition significant. At worst, they could indicate brain displacement or herniation.

Always begin by performing a thorough neurologic assessment. This gives you a baseline for all future assessments. Then, reassess your patient at regular intervals, depending on his condition. (To learn how to do a neurologic assessment, read the *Nursing80* PHOTOBOOK *Assessing Your Patients.*)

Document your observations thoroughly. Avoid using words and phrases that may be interpreted several ways; for example, "Patient is semicomatose." Instead, be specific. Say something like: "Patient is unresponsive to verbal stimuli, and responds to pain by moving his head." Remember, the next health-care professional who looks at your patient will judge the patient's progress—or lack of it—by comparing her observations with yours. Make your notes as detailed as possible.

Notify the doctor if you observe change or deterioration indicating rising ICP in one or more of these areas:
• *Level of consciousness.* If the patient's conscious, note whether he's alert and oriented. Can you get his attention easily? Does he respond intelligibly to your questions? Can he recognize family members? Does he know where he is? Is he more restless or more lethargic than usual?
• *Vital signs.* Since elevated ICP may affect vital signs regulators in the patient's brain, changes in temperature, blood pressure, respiratory patterns, and pulse may signal trouble. Stay alert.
• *Pupillary activity.* Check the patient's pupils periodically. How widely are they dilated? Are they dilated equally? Do they respond to light? Is reaction to light slower in one eye than in the other?
• *Motor and sensory function.* Assess the patient's extremities for sensation, strength, and reflexes. For example, can he feel touch or pressure on his arm? Can he squeeze your fingers with his hand? Can he lift his foot? Does he have blurred or double vision? Does he have the doll's eye reflex? If he's unconscious, does he exhibit decerebrate or decorticate posturing? (For details on these postures, as well as the doll's eye reflex, see the next page.)

Important: Whenever you assess your patient, check responses on *both* sides of his body. Remember, if elevated ICP affects only one hemisphere of the patient's brain, only one side of his body may show signs of distress.

Recognizing brain stem involvement

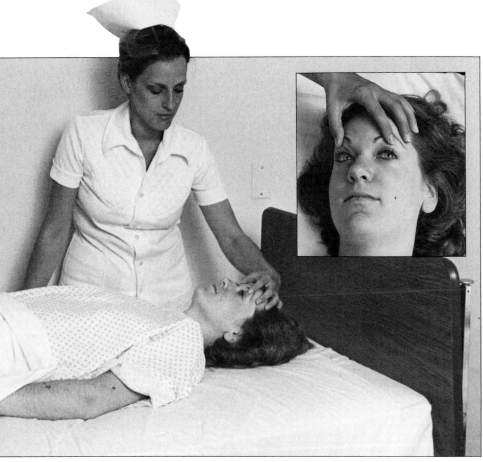

1 When your patient's condition affects her brain stem, diminishing her level of consciousness, she may display certain abnormal reflexes: the doll's eye reflex, decorticate posturing, or decerebrate posturing. If you see one or more of these reflexes, notify the doctor. Your patient's condition may be deteriorating. Here's how to recognize them.

To test for the doll's eye reflex, hold your patient's eyelids open. If her eyes appear fixed and staring straight ahead, quickly (but gently) turn her head to one side. If your patient exhibits the doll's eye reflex, her eyes *won't* move in the direction you turn her head, as you'd expect them to. Instead, they'll remain fixed and in their original position, as shown in the inset.

If brain stem involvement is severe, you may see other abnormal reactions as well. For example, only one eye may move, or each eye may move in a different direction.

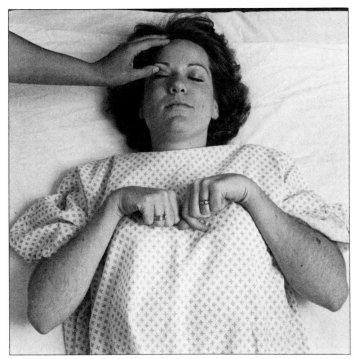

2 With any brain stem involvement, your patient may respond to pain or touch by decorticate posturing, as shown here. As you can see, this patient's arms are in full flexion on her chest. In addition, her legs may be extended stiffly.

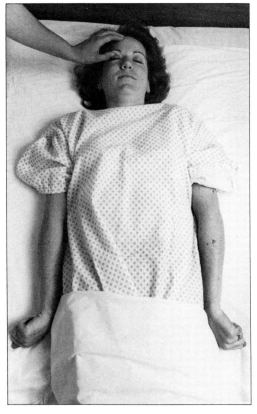

3 Here we see decerebrate posturing. Note how the patient's arms are stiffly extended, with the palms outward. Her legs may also be extended.

Decerebrate posturing suggests even greater pressure on the brain stem than decorticate posturing. But if the pressure's severe, the patient may fail to respond at all to touch or pain. Consider this an extremely ominous sign.

Important: Remember, a motor impairment like hemiplegia may produce *unilateral* reflexes. Consider these as significant as bilateral ones.

Intracranial monitors

Caring for the patient on intracranial pressure (ICP) monitoring

When you care for a critically ill patient, you probably try to schedule many nursing care procedures together. In this way, you avoid disturbing him repeatedly.

But the patient suffering from high intracranial pressure (ICP) needs special consideration. Many nursing procedures—even routine ones, like repositioning—tend to raise a patient's ICP. A cluster of nursing procedures done all at once may spike his ICP and produce menacing A waves. That's why you should do your best to schedule stressful procedures apart.

Read this chart carefully. You'll see how certain stresses can endanger your patient. Then, you'll learn how to minimize them—or avoid them altogether.

Nursing order	Rationale	Additional considerations
Maintain oxygenation; avoid hypoxia and/or hypercapnia	• A CO_2 excess and/or O_2 deficit in arterial blood stimulates cerebral vasodilation, increasing cerebral blood flow (CBF). • Increasing CBF raises ICP.	• Maintain a patent airway. • Monitor arterial blood gas (ABG) measurements closely. • If the doctor orders, hyperventilate the patient before suctioning, to minimize CO_2 accumulation during the procedure. • Limit suctioning to 10 to 15 seconds.
Maintain venous outflow from the brain	• Obstructions to venous outflow increase capillary pressure and diminish absorption of CSF. • Decreased outflow permits CO_2 and lactic acid to accumulate in the brain. Both stimulate cerebral vasodilation. • ICP rises when venous outflow slows. • As a response to rising ICP, blood pressure may drop, causing cerebral ischemia.	• Do not place patient flat or in Trendelenburg position, unless the doctor orders. Instead, elevate the patient's head 30°, or as the doctor orders. • Position the patient's head and neck directly above his midline to avoid compressing a jugular vein. • If the patient has an endotracheal tube in place, make sure the tape securing it doesn't compress the jugular veins.
Avoid increasing intrathoracic or intra-abdominal pressure (Valsalva maneuver)	• Added thoracic or abdominal pressure can spike ICP by increasing pressure on central veins.	• Do not place patient in Trendelenburg position, even for insertion of jugular or subclavian vein catheter, unless the doctor orders. • Do not ask the patient to execute a Valsalva maneuver, even during insertion of jugular or subclavian vein catheter. Instead, expect the doctor to minimize the danger of air embolism by using a syringe to apply suction to the catheter. • Do your best to prevent the patient from using the Valsalva maneuver during bowel movements. Keep his stools soft with an appropriate diet and/ or stool softeners. However, do not administer an enema. • Prevent isometric muscular contractions. Assist your patient when he sits up, and instruct him not to push against the bed's footboard. But if the doctor orders, encourage the patient to perform passive range-of-motion (ROM) exercises. • Ask the patient to exhale when you turn him. • Avoid hip flexion. When catheterizing a female patient, for example, flex her legs as little as possible.
Prevent wide or sudden variations in systemic blood pressure	• Normally, autoregulation maintains cerebral perfusion pressure (CPP) at a level equal to mean systemic arterial pressure (MSAP) minus ICP. But autoregulation may fail when ICP is high. If so, CPP fluctuates with systemic blood pressure. Thus, an increase in systemic arterial pressure (SAP) increases cerebral blood flow (CBF), elevates ICP, and worsens cerebral edema. • Conversely, decreases in SAP may produce cerebral ischemia, allowing CO_2 and lactic acid to accumulate.	• Use blood pressure and ICP monitors to evaluate the effect of stressful nursing procedures; for example, endotracheal tube insertion, suctioning, chest physiotherapy, and repositioning. Document your findings carefully. • Minimize pain with a sedative or topical anesthetic, as ordered by the doctor. • If ordered, use muscle relaxants to calm a combative patient during procedures like endotracheal tube insertion. However, avoid using restraints, unless ordered by the doctor. • Rapid eye movement (REM) stages of sleep may cause a rise in ICP. Never perform stress-producing procedures during REM sleep.
Prevent systemic infection (sepsis)	• Sepsis may produce increased cardiac output and vasodilation, increasing CBF.	• Maintain scrupulous sterile technique when changing equipment or the patient's dressing. • Obtain a CSF sample daily, and send it to the lab for culturing. *Note:* Before obtaining a CSF sample from the drainage bag, remove the bag and tubing and replace them with sterile ones. Never open the CSF drainage bag while it's attached to the patient, or you risk infecting him. • Notify doctor promptly if the patient's temperature increases. • Change the equipment and the dressing on the insertion site daily.

How elevated ICP is treated

As you know, intracranial pressure (ICP) monitoring simply *measures* ICP. To *reduce* ICP, the doctor will probably choose one of these treatments. Study this chart to learn how each one works, and how you can help.

Treatment	What it does	Nursing considerations
Administration of osmotic diuretics; for example, mannitol (Osmitrol*) by I.V. drip or bolus	• Reduces cerebral edema, shrinking intracranial contents	• Monitor fluids and electrolytes (including osmolality) closely. Treatment may cause rapid dehydration. • Watch for a rebound rise in ICP from treatment. • To prevent crystallization, always store mannitol in a closed container under a 15 watt light bulb.
Administration of I.V. steroids; for example, dexamethasone (Decadron*)	• Lowers sodium and water concentration in the brain, reducing cerebral edema	• As ordered, give steroids with antacids orally and cimetidine (Tagamet*) orally or I.V., to prevent peptic ulcers. • Watch for GI bleeding.
Withdrawal of cerebrospinal fluid (CSF) via ventricular catheter or lumbar puncture (spinal tap)	• Reduces CSF volume	• If the doctor uses a ventricular catheter, prevent sepsis by changing the tubing and drainage bag with each CSF withdrawal. • If the doctor performs a lumbar puncture, watch the patient closely for signs of neurologic deterioration (see pages 44 and 45). The sudden drop in ICP may allow the brain to herniate into CSF space.
Restriction of fluid	• Reduces cerebral edema and shrinks brain size, provided the brain's not diseased	• Monitor fluids and electrolytes (including osmolality) closely. Dehydration below 325 Osm may have little therapeutic value. • Maintain fluid restrictions, according to the doctor's orders. (He'll probably restrict an adult patient to 1,200 to 1,500 ml/day.) • Document the patient's fluid intake accurately. *Remember:* Include all I.V. medications in your calculations.
Hyperventilation with hand-held resuscitator or ventilator	• Helps blow off CO_2, constricting blood vessels and reducing cerebral blood flow	• Monitor arterial blood gas measurements. Notify the doctor if CO_2 continues to rise. He may want to increase the rate of ventilation.
Administration of barbiturates to induce coma; for example, phenobarbital (Luminal*)	• Decreases cerebral metabolic rate; decreases cerebral blood flow	• Monitor vital signs, especially respirations, regularly. • Give barbiturates as ordered. *Remember:* You'll have difficulty assessing your patient's mental status when he's receiving barbiturates.
Surgical removal of skull bone flap	• Provides room for swollen brain to expand	• Keep site clean and dry to prevent infection. • Maintain sterile technique when redressing the site.

*Available in the United States and in Canada.

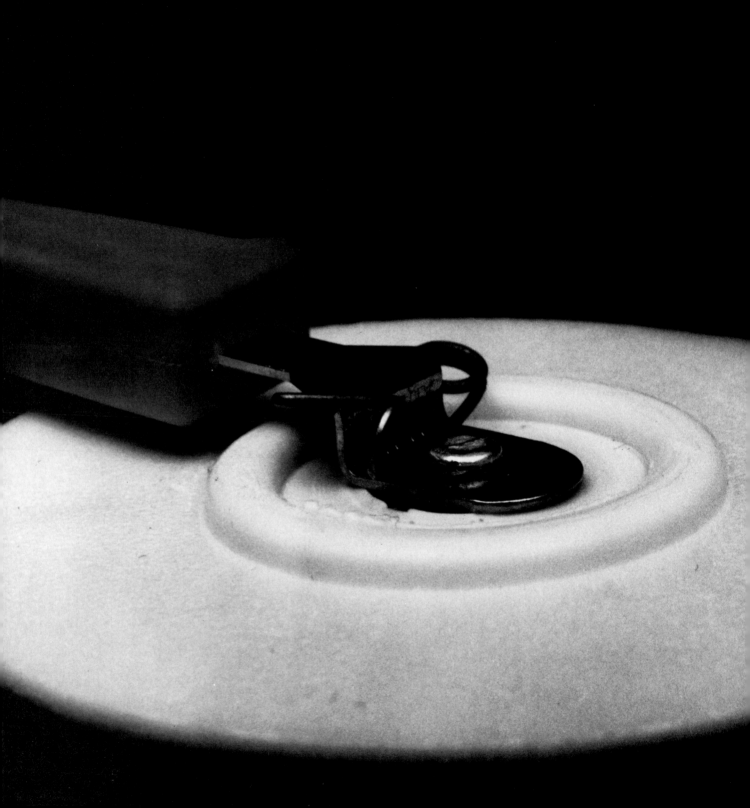

Measuring Cardiac Conduction

Cardiac monitors

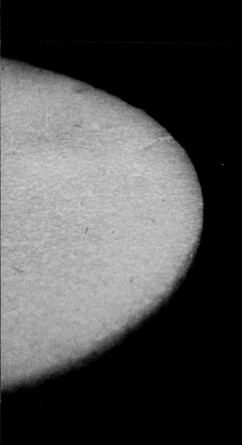

Cardiac monitors

You'll use a cardiac monitor when the doctor wants to learn about your patient's heart conduction. Do you know how a cardiac monitor works? Put simply, electrodes are applied to your patient's chest. These electrodes then pick up the electrical impulses generated by his heart and send them to the monitor. Then, the monitor translates these impulses into a waveform that you or another healthcare professional can analyze to interpret your patient's cardiac condition.

What type of monitor is right for your patient? In the next few pages, we'll examine three monitoring systems:
• Hardwire (or continuous) monitoring for around-the-clock monitoring of the patient on bed rest
• Telemetry monitoring for around-the-clock monitoring of the convalescing patient
• Holter monitoring for short-term monitoring of the ambulatory patient.

Understanding monitors

Not all monitors are exactly alike, but virtually every monitor features most of the components shown here. If your monitor's instrumentation panel differs significantly from this one, check the operator's manual for instructions.

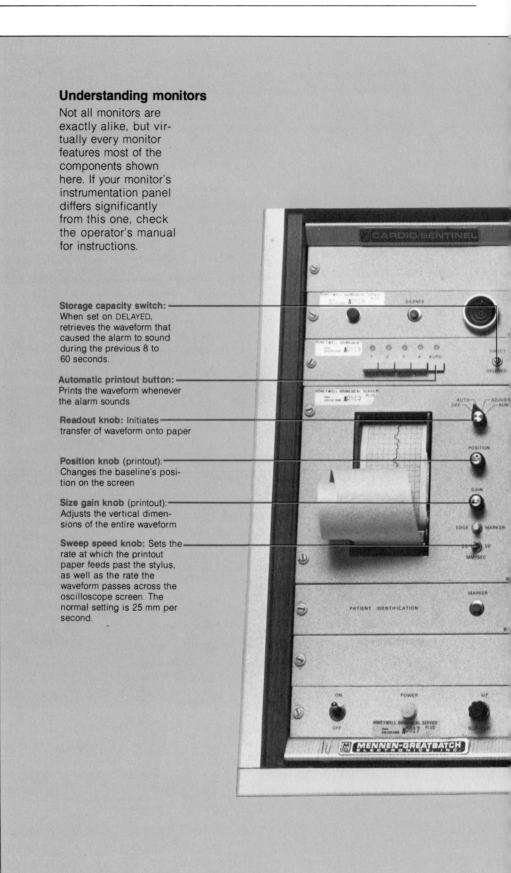

Storage capacity switch: When set on DELAYED, retrieves the waveform that caused the alarm to sound during the previous 8 to 60 seconds.

Automatic printout button: Prints the waveform whenever the alarm sounds

Readout knob: Initiates transfer of waveform onto paper

Position knob (printout): Changes the baseline's position on the screen

Size gain knob (printout): Adjusts the vertical dimensions of the entire waveform

Sweep speed knob: Sets the rate at which the printout paper feeds past the stylus, as well as the rate the waveform passes across the oscilloscope screen. The normal setting is 25 mm per second.

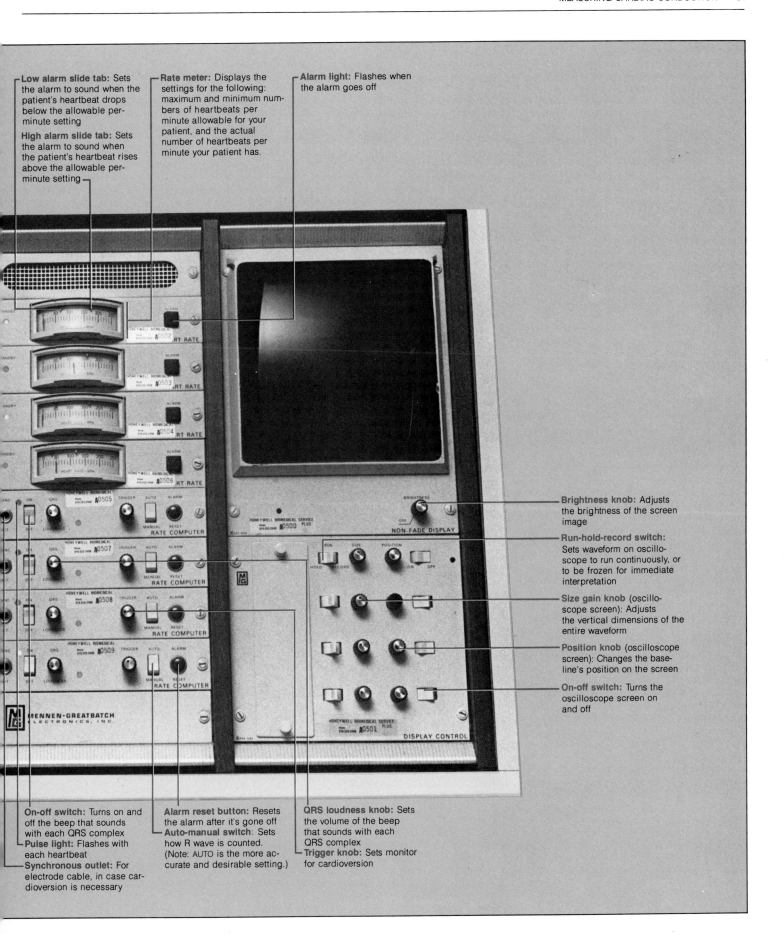

Low alarm slide tab: Sets the alarm to sound when the patient's heartbeat drops below the allowable per-minute setting

High alarm slide tab: Sets the alarm to sound when the patient's heartbeat rises above the allowable per-minute setting

Rate meter: Displays the settings for the following: maximum and minimum numbers of heartbeats per minute allowable for your patient, and the actual number of heartbeats per minute your patient has.

Alarm light: Flashes when the alarm goes off

Brightness knob: Adjusts the brightness of the screen image

Run-hold-record switch: Sets waveform on oscilloscope to run continuously, or to be frozen for immediate interpretation

Size gain knob (oscilloscope screen): Adjusts the vertical dimensions of the entire waveform

Position knob (oscilloscope screen): Changes the baseline's position on the screen

On-off switch: Turns the oscilloscope screen on and off

On-off switch: Turns on and off the beep that sounds with each QRS complex

Pulse light: Flashes with each heartbeat

Synchronous outlet: For electrode cable, in case cardioversion is necessary

Alarm reset button: Resets the alarm after it's gone off

Auto-manual switch: Sets how R wave is counted. (Note: AUTO is the more accurate and desirable setting.)

QRS loudness knob: Sets the volume of the beep that sounds with each QRS complex

Trigger knob: Sets monitor for cardioversion

Cardiac monitors

Understanding electrodes

Whichever type of continuous cardiac monitoring system you use, each employs electrodes and lead wires. An electrode is an electrically conductive disc or needle. When you apply it to your patient's chest, it can detect the electrical impulses that his heart generates. The lead wires, connected to the electrodes, transmit these impulses to the cardiac monitor.

You won't find it difficult to apply electrodes to your patient's skin, but you must do it correctly or you'll distort his EKG readings. Begin your understanding of the procedure by learning about the three basic types of electrodes:

• *Metal disc electrode.* This type of electrode is applied to skin that has first been prepared with a special jelly that conducts electrical impulses. The metal disc electrode poses three problems: first, the conductive jelly can dry and will require replacing; second, the metal disc can pick up extraneous electrical activity; and third, the metal disc can cause the patient discomfort.

• *Needle electrode.* This type of electrode avoids the problems you can encounter by using conductive jelly, because no jelly is needed. But needle electrodes are very difficult to stabilize, so they're rarely used.

• *Floating electrode.* This widely used electrode (pictured below) comes with a pre-jellied cushion between the electrode plate and the patient's skin. You'll find that a floating electrode is easy to apply, can remain on the patient's skin for days, and can conduct electrical impulses without distortion. Because this type is used so extensively, we'll feature it on the following pages.

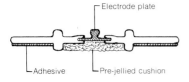

Electrode plate

Adhesive — Pre-jellied cushion

How to apply an electrode

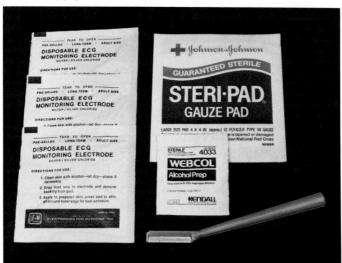

1 *Correct electrode application is a crucial part of the monitoring procedure. But it's not difficult, if you follow these steps.*

Begin by assembling this equipment: three disposable floating electrodes, an alcohol swab, a safety razor with blade, and a sterile gauze pad. Bring these items to your patient's bedside. Explain the procedure to your patient, and answer all his questions. Make sure he realizes that the electrodes can't give him an electric shock.

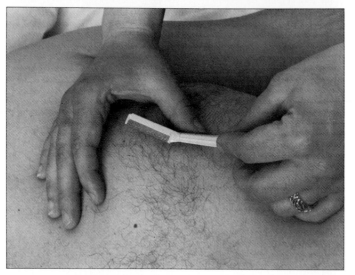

2 Then, ask his permission to shave the small area on his chest where you'll apply the electrodes. Explain that the electrodes will adhere better to skin that's been shaved. They'll also be easier to remove.

Note: The sites you shave are determined by the doctor's lead choice. For more on leads, and their placement, turn the page.

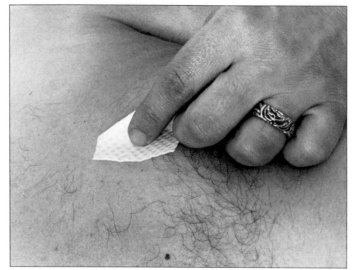

3 Prep the shaven area with an alcohol swab. Let the patient's skin dry completely before continuing.

4 Now, abrade his skin slightly with the gauze pad or some other rough material. Some floating electrodes come with a rough patch to rub on the skin.

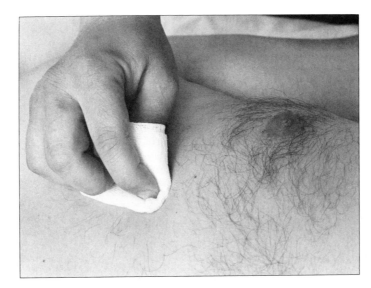

5 Peel off the paper backing on an electrode. As you do, avoid touching the adhesive unnecessarily. Check the sponge pad in the center of the electrode to see if it's still moist with conductive jelly. If the sponge pad's dry, discard the electrode and replace it.

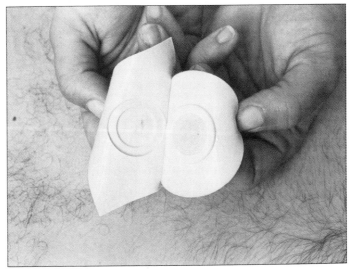

6 Place the electrode, adhesive side down, on the intended site. Then, ensure a good seal by applying pressure, beginning at the center of the electrode and moving outward. If you apply pressure by starting on one side and moving to the other, you could force out some of the conductive jelly from under the electrode, impairing conduction.

Follow this same procedure for applying the remaining electrodes.

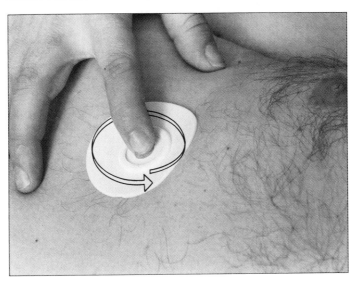

Understanding EKG waves

Every beat of the heart depends on an electrical process called polarization. The first step of this electrical process, *depolarization,* stimulates the muscles in the heart wall. During the second step, *repolarization,* the muscles relax. Translate this process into a waveform, and you have an electrocardiogram (EKG). Here's what a normal EKG looks like:

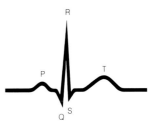

The various points of the wave have been arbitrarily labeled P,Q,R,S, and T. The P wave is the result of atrial depolarization. The QRS wave reflects ventricular depolarization. The T wave represents ventricular repolarization. (The wave reflecting atrial repolarization is usually obscured by the stronger QRS wave.)

Learn how to recognize and understand the waveform of a normal heartbeat. Then you can compare your patient's waveform to it and identify possible abnormalities. For example, suppose his P wave is abnormally shaped. You can surmise that the patient has some condition affecting the depolarization of his heart's atria. Of course, *diagnosing* the condition is the doctor's job. But since you're responsible for maintaining the monitoring system and notifying the doctor of abnormalities, you should be familiar with the basics of reading EKGs. The information on page 66 will help.

Cardiac monitors

How to position electrodes for hardwire monitoring

To perform a complete electrocardiogram, you'll arrange the electrodes to obtain 12 different leads. Each lead monitors a special aspect of the electrical activity of the heart. The doctor will choose the lead, depending on what part of the heart he wants to monitor. There are three standard limb leads (I, II, III), three augmented limb leads (AVR, AVL, and AVF), and six chest leads (V1 through V6).

Suppose you're using a monitor with three electrodes. You can establish the three standard limb leads and the three augmented limb leads without difficulty, because each arrangement requires only three electrodes. But you'll need five electrodes to establish the V1 through V6 chest leads. So, when you have a three-

Type	Lead	Electrode placement	
Three-electrode monitor	Lead II	Positive (+): left side of chest, lowest palpable rib, midclavicular Negative (−): right shoulder, below clavicular hollow Ground (G): left shoulder, below clavicular hollow	
	MCL1	Positive (+): right sternal border, lowest palpable rib Negative (−): left shoulder, below clavicular hollow Ground (G): right shoulder, below clavicular hollow	
	MCL6	Positive (+): left side of chest, lowest palpable rib, midclavicular Negative (−): left shoulder, below clavicular hollow Ground (G): right shoulder, below clavicular hollow	
Five-electrode monitor	V1 through V6	Positive (+): left side of chest, just below lowest palpable rib Negative (−): right shoulder, midclavicular Ground (G): right side of chest, just below lowest palpable rib Inactive (I): left shoulder, midclavicular Chest V1: fourth intercostal space to right of sternum Chest V2: fourth intercostal space to left of sternum Chest V3: halfway between V2 and V4 Chest V4: fifth intercostal space, midclavicular, left side Chest V5: halfway between V4 and V6 Chest V6: fifth intercostal space at midaxillary line	

electrode monitor, use the modified chest leads described in this chart instead. These leads yield readings similar to the V_1 and V_6 chest leads but require only three electrodes. Modified chest leads are abbreviated as MCL_1 and MCL_6. You'll find that for general monitoring on a three-electrode monitor, you'll use standard limb lead II, MCL_1, and MCL_6.

You can do more precise cardiac monitoring with a five-electrode monitor. Such a monitor is capable of recording all 12 leads without distortion or modification. Study this chart to learn about the leads you'll use with both three-electrode and five-electrode monitors.

Purpose	Advantages	Disadvantages	Waveform
• Identifies atrial and ventricular arrhythmias	• Clear P wave • Tall, distinct R wave	• Can't distinguish between right or left bundle branch blocks	
• Identifies atrial and ventricular arrhythmias • Identifies complete and incomplete right bundle branch blocks • Identifies ventricular conduction	• Positive electrode placement doesn't interfere with auscultation or defibrillation	• R wave depressed or of insufficient voltage • Not useful in detection of left bundle branch block or left ventricular hypertrophy	
• Identifies ventricular arrhythmias • Detects left bundle branch block • Replaces MCL_1 if that arrangement can't be used	• Good R wave	• Difficult to detect right bundle branch block • Poor visualization of atrial and arrhythmic activity	
• Obtains a precise, multiplaned view of the heart's activity • Detects hemiblocks	• Standard and augmented leads obtained by turning on a monitor switch, instead of moving an electrode	• Two more electrodes are attached to the patient's chest	LEAD V1 LEAD V4 LEAD V2 LEAD V5 LEAD V3 LEAD V6

Cardiac monitors

Using a hardwire monitor

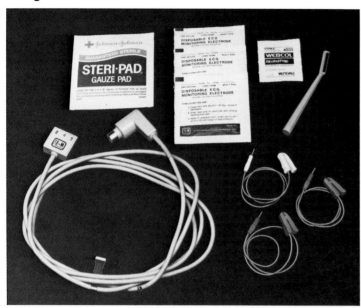

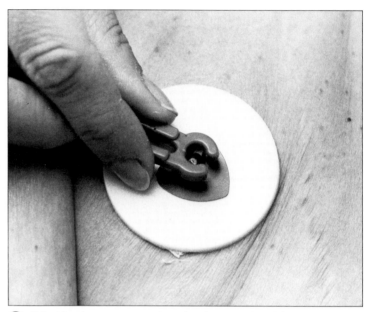

1 *Seventy-five-year-old Violet Penski has suffered a myocardial infarction and has been admitted to the CCU where you work. The doctor wants Mrs. Penski's heart monitored continuously, so he's ordered hardwire monitoring. Do you know how to initiate this type of monitoring? This photostory will show you, using a three-electrode monitor.*

Begin by assembling this equipment: three disposable floating electrodes, an alcohol swab, a sterile 4" x 4" gauze pad, a razor (if needed), three lead wires, and a lead wire receptacle and cable. You'll find the monitor waiting for use at your patient's bedside.

3 What lead arrangement has the doctor ordered for the monitoring? Check the chart shown on the preceding pages to see where to apply the electrodes for that lead. Then, after you apply them—using the procedure on pages 52 and 53—attach the lead wires to the three electrodes, as the nurse is doing here.

How can you tell which lead wires attach to which electrodes? If your lead wires are marked +, −, G (and R if you're using a four-electrode monitor), follow the directions in the chart on the preceding pages.

But what if your lead wires are coded RA, LA, LL, and, with five-electrode monitors, RL and V (sometimes labeled C)? Then, mentally divide your patient's chest into quadrants. Attach the RA lead wire to the electrode positioned nearest to the patient's right arm. Attach the RL lead wire to the electrode nearest to the patient's right leg, and so on.

If your lead wires are color-coded, consult the operator's manual for instructions.

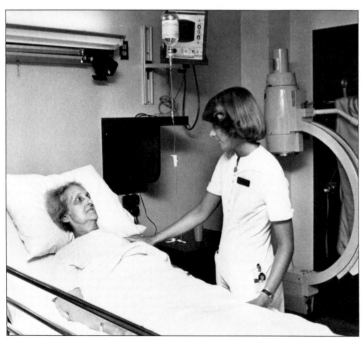

2 Tell the patient what you're going to do and why. Answer any questions she has before continuing the procedure.

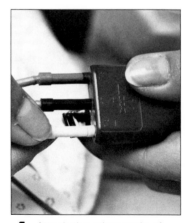

4 Attach the other ends of the lead wires to the lead wire receptacle on the electrode cable. Make sure each lead wire is in its correct outlet.

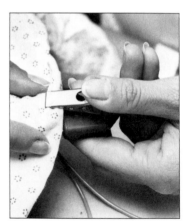

5 Fasten the lead wire receptacle to the patient's gown. This prevents undue stress on the lead wires when the patient moves.

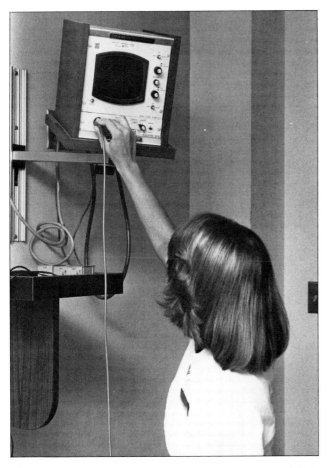

6 Now, securely attach the lead wire receptacle cable to the bedside monitor.

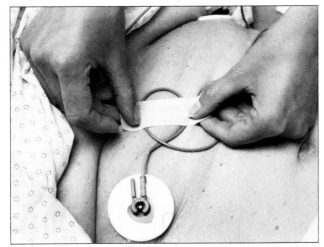

7 Form a stress loop in each lead wire, and tape it to the patient's skin, as shown here. Leave enough slack between the electrode and the stress loop to allow for patient movement without straining the electrode connection. *Important:* Is your patient allergic to adhesive tape? Use nonallergenic tape instead.

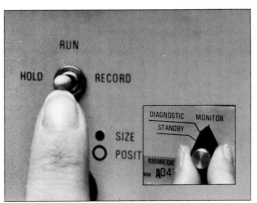

8 Turn the HOLD-RUN-RECORD switch to RUN. [Inset] Then, turn the mode switch from STANDBY to MONITOR. Expect a tracing to appear in about 20 seconds.

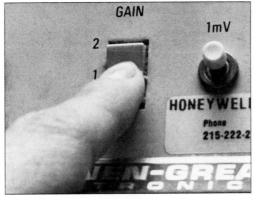

9 Set the GAIN switch to 1 or 2, depending on the size of the QRS complex you're getting. Don't make the QRS complex so tall that it barely fits on the oscilloscope screen.

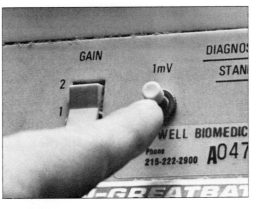

10 Next, calibrate the monitor by pressing the button marked 1MV or CAL, depending on the make of your equipment. This will produce a 1 millivolt high waveform on the oscilloscope screen. Is the R spike of the QRS complex higher than the 1 millivolt waveform? If not, adjust the GAIN setting so it is.

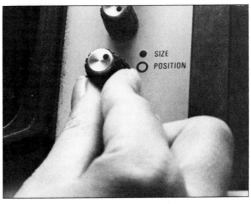

11 Then, adjust the position of the waveform so it's centered on the oscilloscope screen.

Cardiac monitors

Using a hardwire monitor continued

12 If your monitoring system uses a central console, examine it, as the nurse is doing here. Find the group of controls on the console face that corresponds to the controls on the bedside monitor.

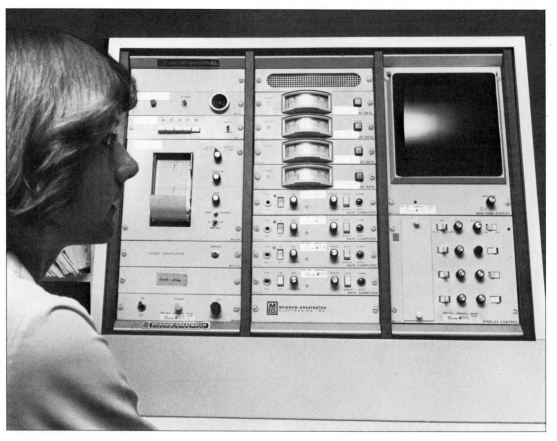

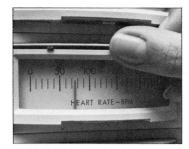

13 Then, touching only those controls, set the HIGH alarm at 120 beats per minute and the LOW alarm at 50 beats per minute, unless the doctor orders otherwise.

If your monitoring system has only bedside units, use the procedure just described to set the HIGH and the LOW alarms on the bedside monitor. Then, go on to the next step.

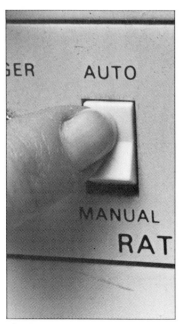

14 Set the heart rate alarm to AUTO, so it'll sound whenever the patient's heart rate goes above or below the limits you've set.

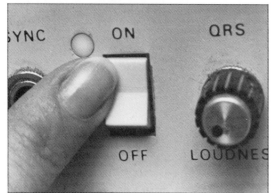

15 Now, check to see if each QRS complex on the oscilloscope screen is being counted by the monitor. First, turn the audible QRS signal on. It will sound with each QRS complex counted. You can also tell by watching the rate light. If the audible alarm doesn't sound, or the rate light doesn't blink with each complex, increase the GAIN setting until the QRS complex is of sufficient height to trigger the audible alarm and the rate light every time. *Note:* Don't make the QRS complex so tall that it interferes with other waveforms on the console's oscilloscope screen. Adjust the size and position of the waveform as you did on the bedside monitor.

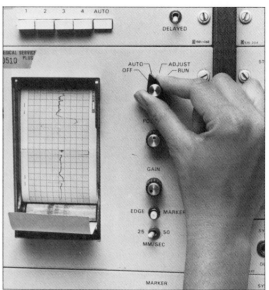

16 Turn the recorder to AUTO and the SWEEP to 25 mm/sec. Then, if the patient's heart rate sets off the alarm, the recorder will print as fast as the oscilloscope reading. Finally, check the paper in the recorder. If a refill is needed, add more paper, using the instructions in the operator's manual.

Positioning electrodes for telemetry monitoring

Telemetry requires three basic pieces of equipment: a transmitter with electrodes, relay wires (usually recessed in the hospital ceiling), and a central console. You'll use the electrodes to attach the transmitter to your patient's body. While the patient's freedom of movement isn't as restricted as it would be if he were on hardwire monitoring, it's still somewhat limited with telemetry, because the relay wires can only pick up his heartbeat within a certain distance from the console. That distance, ranging from 50 to 2,000 feet (15.2 to 609.6 m), depends on the make of your equipment.

The telemetry system your hospital uses features either two or three electrodes. As this chart shows, both types can monitor in the standard lead II position or the MCL1 position. But the three-electrode type also allows you to monitor in the MCL6 position. Note the reference electrode in the three-electrode monitor leads. It was designed to reduce distortion and amplify the transmitted EKG signal, but most two-electrode monitors do this effectively without it.

Type	Lead		Electrode placement
Two-electrode monitor	Lead II	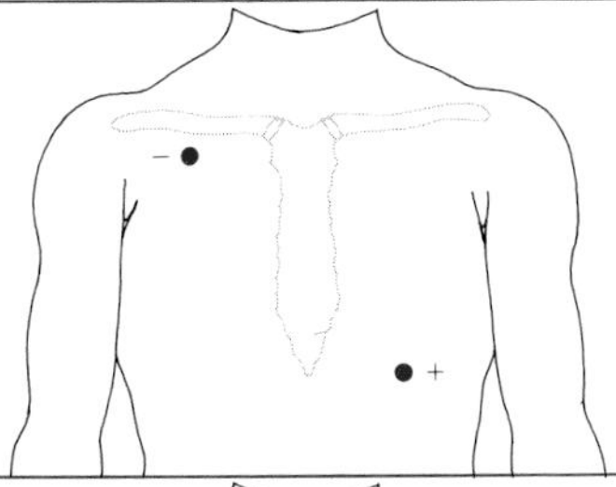	Positive (+): left side of chest, lowest palpable rib, midclavicular Negative (−): right shoulder, below clavicular hollow Ground (G): not applied to patient (built into console)
	MCL1	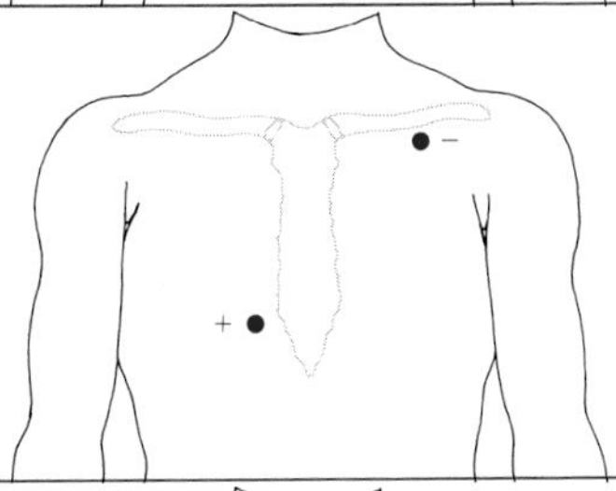	Positive (+): right sternal border, lowest rib Negative (−): left shoulder, below clavicular hollow Ground (G): not applied to patient (built into console)
Three-electrode monitor	Lead II	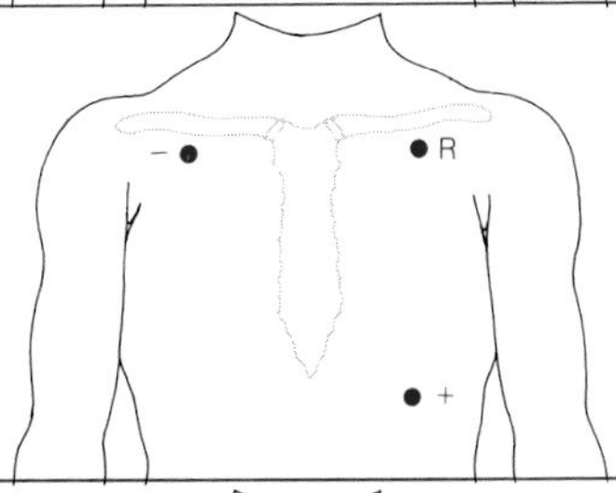	Positive (+): left side of chest, lowest palpable rib, midclavicular Negative (−): right shoulder, below clavicular hollow Ground (G): not applied to patient (built into console) Reference (R): left shoulder, below clavicular hollow
	MCL1	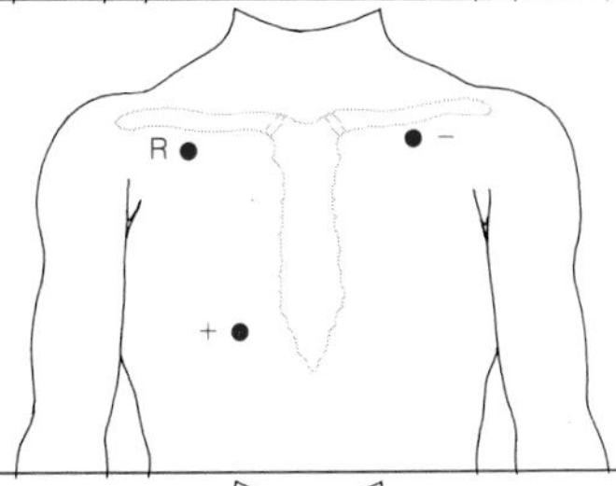	Positive (+): right sternal border, lowest palpable rib Negative (−): left shoulder, below clavicular hollow Ground (G): not applied to patient (built into console) Reference (R): right shoulder, below clavicular hollow
	MCL6	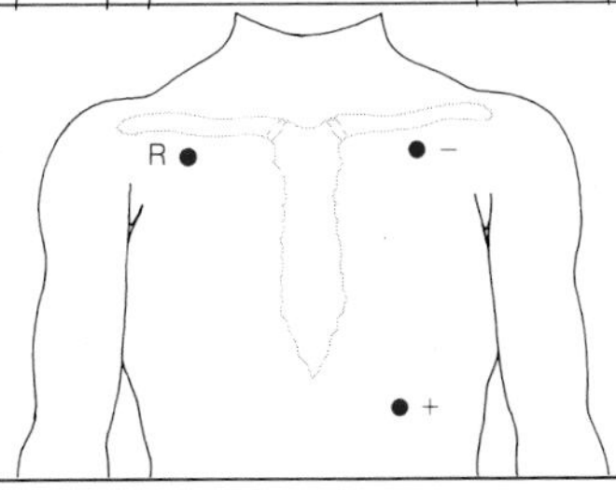	Positive (+): left side of chest, lowest palpable rib, midclavicular Negative (−): left shoulder, below clavicular hollow Ground (G): not applied to patient (built into console) Reference (R): right shoulder, below clavicular hollow

Cardiac monitors

Using telemetry

1 *Hans Wilheim, a 48-year-old house painter, suffered an anterior wall myocardial infarction 4 days ago and has been in the CCU ever since. Now, the doctor's ordered him transferred to an intermediate unit, for telemetry monitoring. Do you know how to set up such a monitor? If not, read this photostory.*

Begin by gathering the equipment shown in the inset to use with the telemetry console: a telemetry transmitter, two or three electrodes (depending on the transmitter), a transmitter pouch, and a battery.

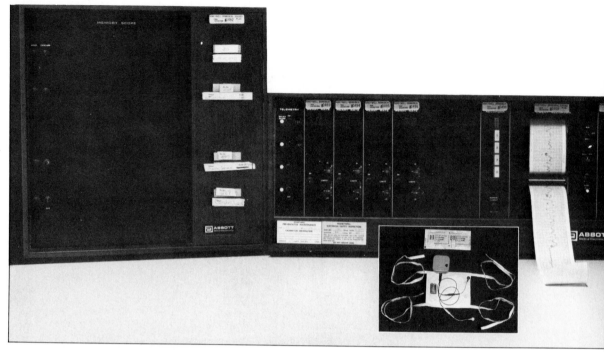

2 Insert the battery into the transmitter, using the polarity markings on the transmitter case.

[Inset] Then, check to see if the battery's working by pushing the test light on the back of the transmitter. If it doesn't light, get a new battery.

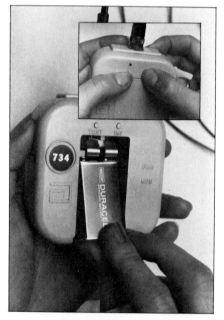

3 Make sure the lead wire cable's securely attached to the transmitter. Now you're ready to talk to the patient.

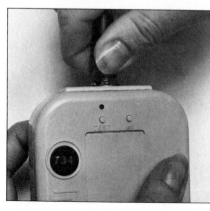

4 Show the transmitter to the patient, and explain how it works. Answer any questions he has before proceeding.

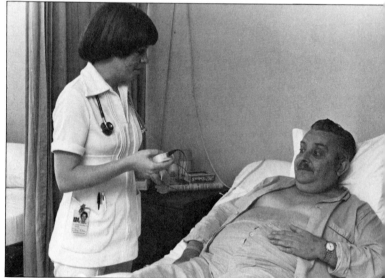

5 Apply the electrodes to his chest, using the procedure explained on pages 52 and 53. Arrange them to establish the lead ordered by the doctor.

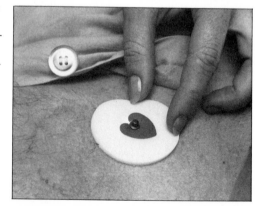

6 Attach lead wires to the electrodes, following the pattern outlined in step 3 on page 56.

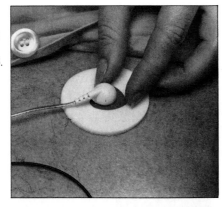

7 Now, place the transmitter into either a cotton pouch provided by the manufacturer, or a handmade pouch provided by the hospital.

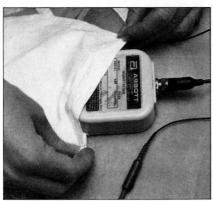

8 Tie the pouch strings around your patient's neck and waist. Make sure the pouch fits snugly, but take care that your patient's not uncomfortable.

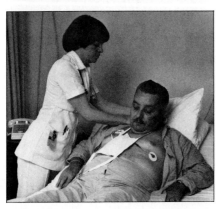

9 Now, go to the monitor's central console, and find the number of your telemetry unit. Turn on its POWER switch.

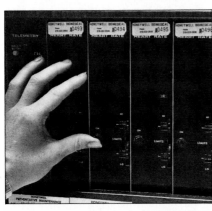

10 Adjust the HIGH alarm and LOW alarm limits, to rates the doctor orders. But first, test the alarms by setting the limits well within the patient's normal rate. When they sound, turn them off, and adjust them as ordered. *Note:* Some telemetry monitors also have an ALARM button, in addition to the high and low settings. If the unit you're using does, test the ALARM button to make sure it's set, too.

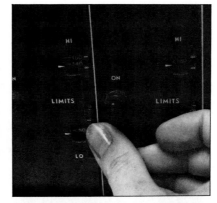

11 Now, turn on the RECORDER button. A printout of waveforms will begin immediately.

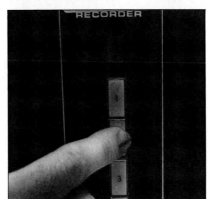

12 Push the CAL button to get a 1 millivolt high waveform. Is the QRS complex greater than 1 millivolt? If not, turn the GAIN CONTROL knob until the waveform height is correct and undistorted.

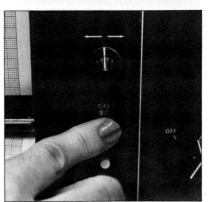

13 Turn the RECORDER button to AUTO so the recorder will automatically begin a printout of the heartbeat if the alarm sounds.

Before you leave the console, make sure everything is properly set, as the nurse is doing here.

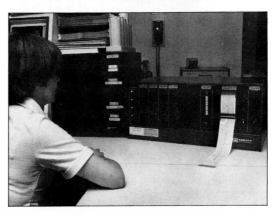

Cardiac monitors

What's Holter monitoring?

You'll use Holter monitoring for the patient:
• recovering from a heart condition.
• taking antiarrhythmic drugs.
• using a pacemaker.
• with possible cardiac symptomatology needing further study.

This portable monitor is designed and equipped to tape record the patient's heartbeat over a 24-hour period. Since it's worn on a belt, it won't interfere with the patient's daily activities. During the 24-hour recording period, the patient keeps a diary of his activities and symptoms. When he returns to the hospital, the tape is run so the recorded waveform can be observed. You can interpret this waveform like any other EKG, and then match the waveform's irregularities to the patient's diary entries to determine the possible causes of these irregularities.

How to position electrodes for Holter monitoring

As a first step, carefully examine the Holter monitor that you'll be using to monitor your patient's heart. Determine whether your hospital uses a single- or a dual-channel recorder unit.

The single-channel recorder has three electrodes and can record only one lead at a time.

In most cases, you'll use standard lead II.

The dual-channel recorder has either four or five electrodes and can record two leads *at the same time*. With this type of recorder, you'll probably monitor standard lead II and MCL1. If your dual-channel recorder has four electrodes, you won't need to apply a ground electrode to the patient, because the ground's built into the monitor. If your dual-channel recorder has five electrodes, the ground you apply to the patient acts in that capacity for both leads. The following chart shows you how these electrodes are placed.

Recorder capacity	Electrode capacity	Electrode arrangement	Electrode placement
Single channel	Three	Standard lead II 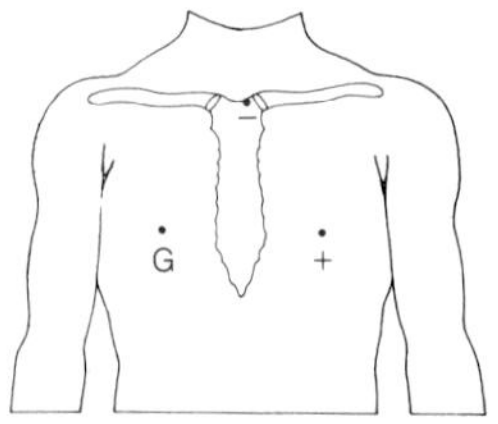	Standard lead II positive (+): over the fifth rib on the left side of the chest Standard lead II negative (−): over the manubrium, the bony area at the top of the sternum Standard lead II ground (G): over the fifth rib on the right side of the chest
Dual channel	Four	Standard lead II and MCL1 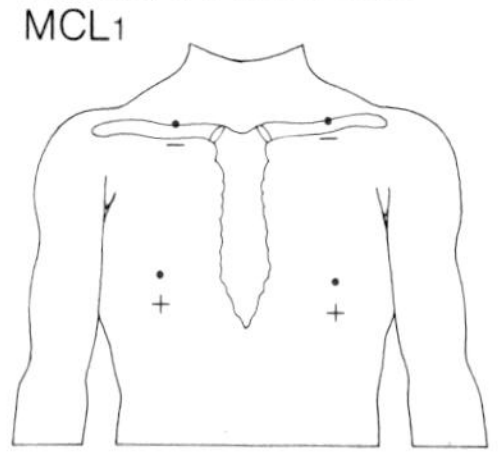	Standard lead II positive (+): over the fifth rib on the left side of the chest Standard lead II negative (−): over the right clavicle at the manubrium Common ground (G): not applied to the patient (built into the monitor) MCL1 positive (+): over the fifth rib on the right side of the chest MCL1 negative (−): over the left clavicle at the manubrium
	Five	Standard lead II and MCL1 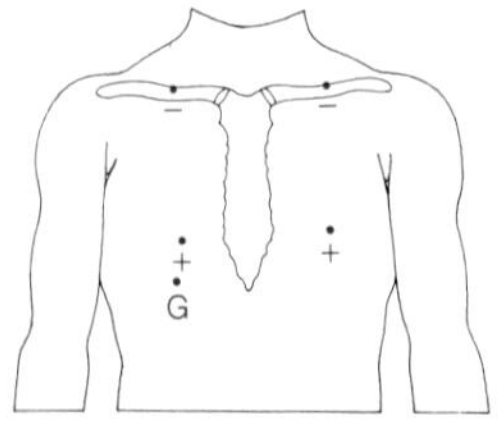	Standard lead II positive (+): over the fifth rib on the left side of the chest Standard lead II negative (−): over the right clavicle at the manubrium Common ground (G): over the sixth rib on the right side of the chest MCL1 positive (+): over the fifth rib on the right side of the chest MCL1 negative (−): over the left clavicle at the manubrium

Using a Holter monitor

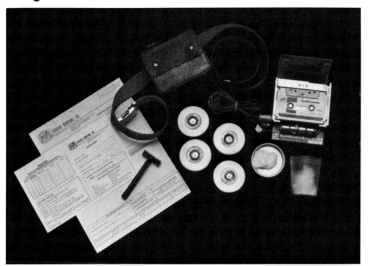

1 *Arthur Barry, a 45-year-old insurance executive, is admitted to your hospital after he complains of severe weakness and dizziness. During this hospitalization, the doctor diagnoses Mr. Barry's condition as ventricular bigeminy, and orders 500 mg of procainamide hydrochloride (Pronestyl*) to be given orally every 6 hours. After 1 week of therapy, Mr. Barry is discharged. But the doctor wants to determine if the medication will continue to be effective when Mr. Barry resumes his regular activities, and if such activities will affect his heart adversely. He orders Holter monitoring, as explained on the opposite page. Do you know how to initiate it?*

Begin by gathering this equipment, in addition to the monitor, its carrying case, and a belt: skin electrodes (three for a single-channel monitor, four or five for a dual-channel monitor), alcohol swabs, a blank cassette tape, a razor and blade, nonallergenic tape (not shown), and a patient diary.

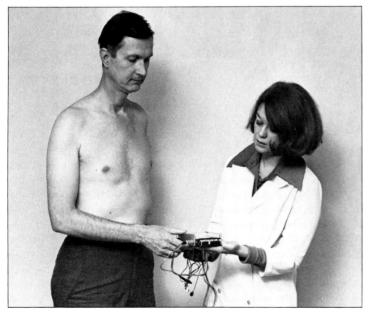

2 Explain the procedure to Mr. Barry. Assure him that the Holter monitor will record his heart rate for 24 hours without interfering with his daily activities.

*Available in the United States and in Canada.

3 Next, prep the skin on his chest, using this procedure: First, determine which leads the doctor wants you to use. Then, shave the area (if necessary), and abrade it with an alcohol swab or gauze pad, using the technique shown on page 53.

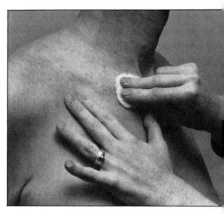

4 Apply the electrodes in the proper positions, using the chart on the opposite page as a guide. In this case, Mr. Barry will be monitored on a dual-channel recorder with the electrodes in the standard lead II and MCL$_1$ position.

Make sure the electrode cable's securely attached to the monitor. [Inset] Then, as your patient holds the monitor and belt, attach lead wires to the electrodes, following the pattern described in step 3 on page 56.

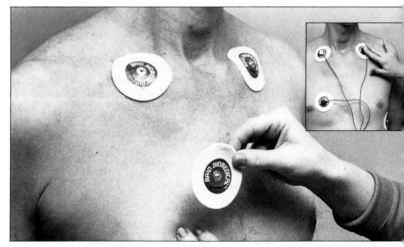

5 Load the cassette recorder with recording tape and turn it on. If the monitor must be calibrated before use, do this by first pushing the calibration button. Then, do one of the following: remove the electrode cable from the Holter monitor, and plug it into a console monitor to get a standard waveform; or let the Holter monitor run for several minutes. Then, pop out the tape, and give it to a trained technician. He'll run the tape on the console monitor to confirm whether or not you're getting an accurate recording. If, in either instance, you're not getting an accurate recording, remove the electrodes and reapply them. Then, make sure the tape cassette is put back in the Holter monitor and the electrode cable is secure before proceeding.

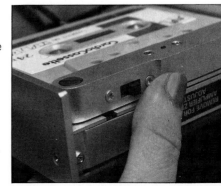

Cardiac monitors

Using a Holter monitor continued

6 Strap the Holter monitor around your patient's waist. Adjust the belt so your patient's comfortable, but don't make it so loose that the monitor's weight pulls on the electrodes.

[Inset 1] Apply nonallergenic tape over each electrode to secure it.

[Inset 2] Then, gather all electrode wires into one loop, and tape that loop to the patient's skin. Make sure you leave enough slack in the loop so the patient's normal movements don't strain the electrode connections.

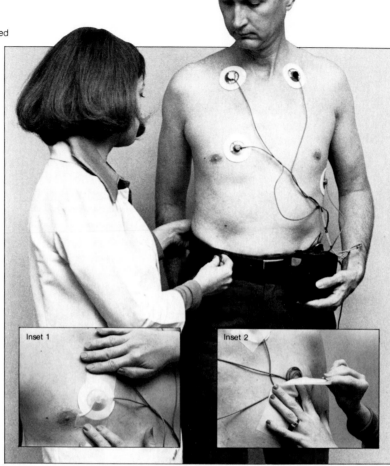

Inset 1

Inset 2

PATIENT TEACHING

Teaching Holter monitoring

Has the doctor ordered Holter monitoring for your patient? Take time to explain this type of monitoring to your patient, and show him how it works. Tell him that the success of the monitoring depends largely on his cooperation. For example, stress how important it is for him to carefully record his activities and symptoms. Finally, give him a blank diary and a copy of the home care aid on the opposite page. Go over the material with him, and answer any questions he has.

7 Explain to the patient that the success of this test depends on his cooperation. Show him the patient diary, and tell him how to complete it. On the opposite page, you'll find a sample Holter diary and a home care aid you can copy and give to your patient.

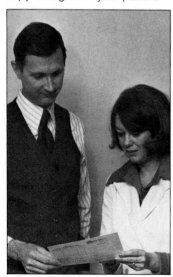

8 When Mr. Barry returns in 24 hours, disconnect the electrodes from his chest, and remove the cassette recorder from the monitor. Then, if you're a qualified technician, insert the recorder into a console, like the one shown here. The console will simultaneously display Mr. Barry's heart rate on the screen and produce a printout of it. This printout can then be interpreted by a cardiologist.

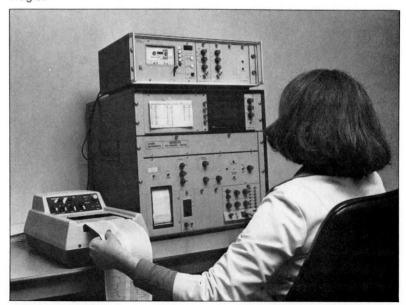

Patient teaching

Home care

What you should know about Holter monitoring

Dear Patient:

Your doctor wants you to wear a Holter monitor to record your heartbeat over the next 24 hours. The information he'll gather from this recording will help him learn how your heart reacts to activity and rest.

To record the electrical impulses from your heart, a nurse or cardiac technician must first apply electrodes to your chest. These electrodes will adhere to your skin like adhesive tape and won't hurt you. Then, she'll attach a portable monitor, which you'll wear on a belt around your waist.

The success of this monitoring depends on your cooperation. For example, while you're wearing the monitor, the doctor wants you to keep track of your activities and symptoms in a patient diary. Keep the diary, as well as a pen or pencil, with you at all times. Jot down the time of day you experience any strong emotions, take medication (including nonprescription drugs), or do any of the following activities: eating, drinking (especially alcohol or caffeinic beverages), moving bowels, urinating, changing posture, engaging in sexual activity, exercising, sleeping.

Also jot down the exact time you had any physical symptoms: for example, dizziness, headache, pain, or mild shortness of breath.

Important: If you experience severe chest pain or shortness of breath, call your doctor, and go to the emergency department of a nearby hospital immediately.

Below is a sample of one patient's diary. Use it as a guideline to help you complete your own diary.

Keep these additional guidelines in mind:
• Do not take the monitor out of its carrying case or meddle with it in any way. Do not disconnect the lead wires or electrodes on your chest.
• Do not let the monitor get wet. Don't shower, bathe, or swim with it on.
• If the light on the monitor flashes on, one of the electrodes on your chest may be loose. Test each one by pressing on the center of it.
• When the 24-hour period is up, return to the hospital with the monitor, and the nurse or technician will remove it. Do not remove it yourself.

TIME	ACTIVITY	SYMPTOMS
11:15 AM	Home from hospital, resting	None
12:00 PM	Prepared and ate lunch, took Pronestyl	None
1:40 PM	Took a walk for 30 minutes	Tired, Legs ached
2:20 PM	Went to bathroom, urinated	Still tired
4:30 PM	Urinated	Dizzy
5:00 PM	Prepared and ate dinner, took Pronestyl	None
6:00 PM	Got up to turn on TV	None
10:10 PM	Urinated	None
10:15 PM	Went to bed	None
2:30 AM	Awoke from sleep, took Pronestyl	Sweating, palpitations
7:20 AM	Got up	Arms heavy
7:25 AM	Urinated	Tired
7:30 AM	Shaved and dressed	Tired
8:00 AM	Prepared and ate breakfast, took Pronestyl	Felt better
10:00 AM	Left for hospital, driving in car	None

Cardiac monitors

EKG interpretation basics

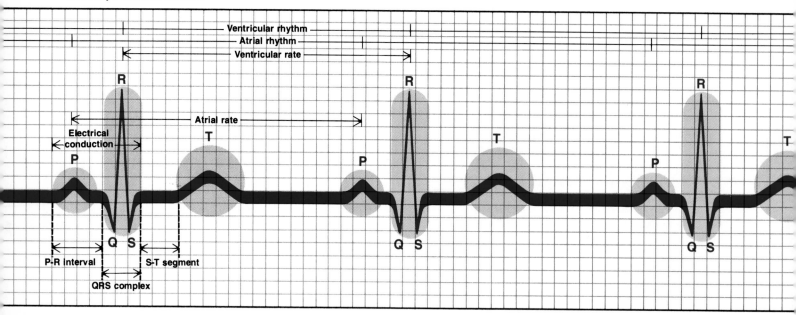

To read an EKG correctly, you must first examine the waveform to gather some basic information from it. Do you know what this basic information is? Read what follows:

● *Heart rhythm:* You can determine whether or not your patient's heart rhythm is regular or irregular by measuring the distance between each wave in a series. To determine atrial rhythm, measure the distance between two P waves, using calipers or a piece of paper. Tighten the calipers, or mark the piece of paper to indicate this distance. Then, using this marked-off distance, compare it with the distances between other P waves on the EKG strip. If the distance between each wave is exactly the same, your patient's atrial rhythm is regular. If the distance varies slightly, his atrial rhythm's slightly irregular. If it varies markedly, his atrial rhythm is considered markedly irregular.

To determine your patient's ventricular rhythm, repeat the entire measuring procedure, using the QRS complexes. Measure from R wave to R wave.

● *Heart rate:* As you probably know, you're measuring only your patient's ventricular heart rate when you take his pulse. But you can measure both his ventricular and atrial heart rates from his EKG. If your patient's heart rhythm is *regular,* follow these steps:

Since the P wave represents atrial activity, you'll use this wave to determine your patient's atrial heart rate. Study two consecutive P waves. Select identical points on each; for example, the waves' starting points or their apex. Then, count the number of squares between these two points.

Each square represents 0.04 seconds. That means that 1,500 squares equal 1 minute. Since you want to find the atrial heart rate per minute, divide 1,500 by the number of squares you counted between P waves. The sum is your patient's atrial heart rate.

Now, repeat the procedure with the QRS complex, measuring from R to R. This will tell you your patient's ventricular heart rate.

If your patient's heart rhythm is *irregular,* follow this procedure instead:

To determine the atrial heart rate, count the number of P waves within the space of 30 large blocks. Since each small block is equal to 0.04 seconds, and it takes five small blocks to make up one large block, each large block equals 0.2 seconds. Thirty large

blocks, therefore, equal 6 seconds. Take the number of P waves you counted within 30 large blocks (6 seconds), and multiply it by 10 to get your patient's atrial rate for 1 minute.

To determine ventricular rate for the patient with an irregular rhythm, repeat the same calculations, this time counting QRS complexes instead.

● *Electrical conduction.* Conduction refers to the time it takes for an electrical impulse originating in the heart's SA node to stimulate ventricular contraction. To determine conduction time, measure the P-R interval and the duration of the QRS complex.

To measure the P-R interval, count the squares between the beginning of the P wave and the beginning of the R wave. Then, multiply this number by 0.04 seconds. The sum represents how long it took an electrical impulse to travel from the heart's SA node through the atrium to the ventricles. The normal time is 0.12 to 0.2 seconds.

Follow the same steps to find the duration of the QRS complex. Count the squares between the beginning of the Q wave and the end of the S wave. Multiply this number by 0.04 seconds to find out how long it took an electrical impulse to pass through the heart's ventricles. The normal time is 0.04 to 0.12 seconds.

● *Configuration and location.* Ask yourself these basic questions to determine the configuration and location of the wave pattern:

Are all the P waves the same size and shape? Do they point in the same direction? Do they precede QRS complexes? Are they all the same distance from the T waves that precede them?

Are all the QRS complexes the same shape and size? Do they point in the same direction? Do they precede T waves? Are they all the same distance from the T waves that follow them?

Are the S-T segments above or below the baseline? Do they line up with the P-R intervals?

Are all the T waves the same shape and size? Do they all point in the same direction? Do they all point in the same direction as the QRS complexes?

Knowing how to gather this basic information will help you learn how to read an EKG. Armed with this information, you can now proceed to the following chart. In it, you'll learn what your observations tell about the electrical activity of your patient's heart.

Making EKG interpretations

Now that you know how to read an EKG, you're one big step closer to understanding the electrical activity of your patient's heart. Although the doctor makes the final diagnosis of your patient's condition, you may get a waveform indicating that your patient requires immediate attention. That's why you should know how to identify basic heart problems, as well. Here's a sampling of EKG findings, accompanied by the appropriate interpretation.

HEART RHYTHM		HEART RATE		ELECTRICAL CONDUCTION	CONFIGURATION	INTERPRETATION
Atrial	Ventricular	Atrial	Ventricular			
Regular	Regular	60 to 100 beats per minute	60 to 100 beats per minute	P-R intervals normal; P wave for every QRS complex	P wave normal; QRS complex normal	Normal sinus rhythm
Regular	Regular	60 beats per minute or less	60 beats per minute or less	P-R intervals normal; P wave for every QRS complex	P wave normal; QRS complex normal	Sinus bradycardia
Regular	Regular	100 to 150 beats per minute	100 to 150 beats per minute	P-R intervals normal; P wave for every QRS complex	P wave normal; QRS complex normal	Sinus tachycardia
Irregular	Irregular	60 to 100 beats per minute	60 to 100 beats per minute	P-R intervals normal; P wave for every QRS complex	P wave normal; QRS complex normal	Sinus arrhythmia
Regular or irregular	Regular or irregular	60 to 100 beats per minute	60 to 100 beats per minute	P-R intervals may vary, but no more than 0.2 seconds; P wave for every QRS complex	P wave variable; QRS complex normal	Wandering pacemaker
Irregular (due to decreased PQRS complex)	Irregular (due to decreased PQRS complex)	Variable	Variable	P-R intervals normal	P wave normal; QRS complex normal	Sinus pause
Irregular (due to premature P waves)	Irregular (due to premature P waves)	Variable	Variable	P-R intervals extended because of premature P waves; P wave for every QRS complex	Premature P waves may be inverted or irregularly shaped	Premature atrial contractions (PAC)
Irregular (due to premature P waves)	Irregular (due to premature P waves)	Variable	Variable	P-R intervals normal when they can be measured; Premature P waves not followed by QRS complex	Premature P waves may be inverted, irregularly shaped, or hidden in QRS complex or T wave ; QRS complex normal	Nonconducted premature atrial contraction
Regular	Regular	150 to 250 beats per minute	150 to 250 beats per minute	P-R intervals normal or prolonged; P wave usually followed by QRS complex	P wave abnormal or inverted but shape stays constant; P wave sometimes merges with T wave; QRS complex normal	Paroxsymal atrial tachycardia (PAT)
Regular	Regular or irregular	250 to 300 beats per minute	Variable	P-R waves constant or variable; QRS complex follows flutter wave, but not all flutter waves are followed by QRS complex	Saw-toothed P waves; QRS complex normal	Atrial flutter
Irregular	Irregular	Over 400 beats per minute	Under 100 beats per minute: controlled Over 100 beats per minute: uncontrolled	P-R intervals can't be measured; P waves indistinct	P wave appears as wavy baseline; QRS complex normal	Atrial fibrillation
Regular (if P wave is visible)	Regular (if P wave is visible)	40 to 60 beats per minute	40 to 60 beats per minute	P-R intervals shorter than normal, when they can be measured; P wave may precede, follow, or be hidden in QRS complex	P wave usually inverted; QRS complex normal	Junctional rhythm

Cardiac monitors

Making EKG interpretations continued

HEART RHYTHM		HEART RATE		ELECTRICAL CONDUCTION	CONFIGURATION	INTERPRETATION
Atrial	Ventricular	Atrial	Ventricular			
Regular or irregular	Regular or irregular	Variable	Variable	Premature P wave shortens P-R intervals; Premature P wave may precede, follow, or be hidden in the QRS complex	Premature P wave otherwise normal; may be inverted or hidden; QRS complex normal	Premature junctional contractions
Regular (if P wave is visible)	Regular	Over 60 beats per minute (if P wave is visible)	Over 60 beats per minute	P-R intervals shorter than normal, if measurable; P wave may precede, follow, or be hidden in the QRS complex	P wave different than sinus P wave, if visible; QRS complex normal	Junctional tachycardia
Regular (if visible)	Regular or irregular	Variable	20 to 40 beats per minute	P-R intervals variable; P wave relationship to QRS complex variable	P wave normal when visible; QRS complex abnormal and widened; T wave usually in opposite direction of QRS complex	Ventricular rhythm
Regular or irregular	Irregular	Variable	Variable	P-R intervals shorter than normal, when they can be measured; P wave relationship to QRS complex variable	P wave constant or variable; QRS complex abnormal and widened; T wave usually in opposite direction of QRS complex	Premature ventricular contraction
Regular (if visible)	Regular	Variable	40 to 100 beats per minute	P-R intervals variable; P wave relationship to QRS complex variable	P wave normal when visible; QRS complex wide and bizarre; T wave opposite of QRS complex	Accelerated ventricular rhythm
Regular	Regular or irregular	Variable	100 to 270 beats per minute	P-R intervals variable; P wave relationship to QRS complex variable	P wave normal when visible; QRS wider than normal, may vary; T wave opposite of QRS complex	Ventricular tachycardia
Not visible	Irregular	Not determinable	Extremely rapid	P-R intervals can't be determined; P wave relationship to QRS complex not visible	P wave not visible; No defined QRS complex	Ventricular fibrillation
Regular (if present)	Not present	Variable	None present	Nonexistent; P wave relationship to QRS complex not visible	P wave normal (if visible); QRS complex not visible	Ventricular standstill
Regular	Regular	Variable with underlying rhythm	Same as atrial	P-R intervals over 0.2 seconds; P wave for every QRS complex	P wave normal; QRS complex normal	First-degree A-V block
Regular	Irregular	Variable, but greater than ventricular	Variable	P-R intervals progressively prolonged; P wave before every QRS complex, but QRS complex may not follow every P wave	P wave normal; QRS complex normal	Second-degree A-V block (Wenckebach)
Regular	Regular, except for pause caused by missing QRS complex	Variable, but greater than ventricular	Variable	P-R intervals normal or prolonged, but consistent; P wave before every QRS complex, but QRS complex may not follow every P wave	P wave normal; QRS complex normal or 0.12 seconds greater than normal	Second-degree A-V block (Mobitz II)
Regular	Regular	Twice that of ventricular	Variable	P-R intervals normal or prolonged, but constant; two P waves for every QRS complex	P wave normal; QRS complex normal	Second-degree A-V block (2:1 conduction)
Regular	Regular	Variable, but greater than ventricular	Variable	P-R intervals variable with no pattern; no relationship between P wave and QRS complex	P wave normal; QRS complex normal or abnormal	Third-degree A-V block

Troubleshooting cardiac monitors

This chart shows you how to troubleshoot the common problems you're apt to encounter while working with cardiac monitors. As you study it, keep in mind that no matter *what* problem arises with the equipment—from a straight line on the oscilloscope screen to a sparking monitor—always examine your patient first.

Problem	Possible causes	Solution
Skin excoriation under electrode	• Patient allergic to electrode adhesive • Electrode left on skin too long	• Remove electrodes and apply nonallergenic electrodes and nonallergenic tape. • Remove electrode, clean site, and reapply electrode at new site.
Broken lead wires or broken cable	• Stress loops not used on lead wires • Cables and lead wires cleaned with alcohol or acetone, causing brittleness	• Replace lead wires and retape them, using stress loops. • Clean cable and lead wires with soapy water instead of alcohol or acetone. *Important:* Do not get cable ends wet.
Wandering baseline	• Patient movement • Improper application of electrodes • Use of nonpolarized electrodes	• Problem disappears when patient relaxes. • Check electrodes and reapply them, if necessary. • Replace electrodes with polarized ones.
Straight line on monitor (not caused by asystole)	• Improper connection of lead wire to either electrode or cable	• Check cable and electrode connections and adjust them, if necessary.
60-cycle interference (fuzzy baseline)	• Electrical interference from other equipment in the room • Improper grounding of patient's bed	• Make sure all electrical equipment is attached to a common ground. Check three-pronged plugs to make sure none of the prongs is loose. • Make sure the bed ground is attached to the room's common ground.
Artifact (waveform interference)	• Patient experiencing seizures, chills, or anxiety • Patient movement • Improper application of electrodes • Electrical short circuit in lead wires or cable • Static electricity interference, from decrease in room humidity	• Notify doctor that the patient's having seizures, and treat patient, as ordered. Keep patient warm and reassured. Spend time with him, and discuss his fears. • Problem should disappear when patient relaxes. • Check electrodes and reapply them, if necessary. • Check electrode jelly and reapply electrode, if necessary. • Replace broken equipment. Use stress loops when applying lead wires. • Regulate room humidity to 40%.
Double-triggering (P wave and QRS complex, or QRS complex and T wave are of equal height)	• Monitor GAIN setting too high, particularly with MCL1 setting	• Reset GAIN setting. If possible, monitor patient on MCL6 or another available lead.
Alarm sounds, but you see no evidence of arrhythmia	• QRS complex too small to register • QRS complex not registering because of MCL1 lead setting • HIGH alarm set too low, or LOW alarm set too high • Artifact (waveform interference)	• Reapply electrodes. • Set GAIN so that the height of the complex is greater than 1 millivolt. • If possible, monitor the patient on MCL6. • Set alarm limits, according to patient's heart rate. • Check electrodes and reapply them, if necessary.

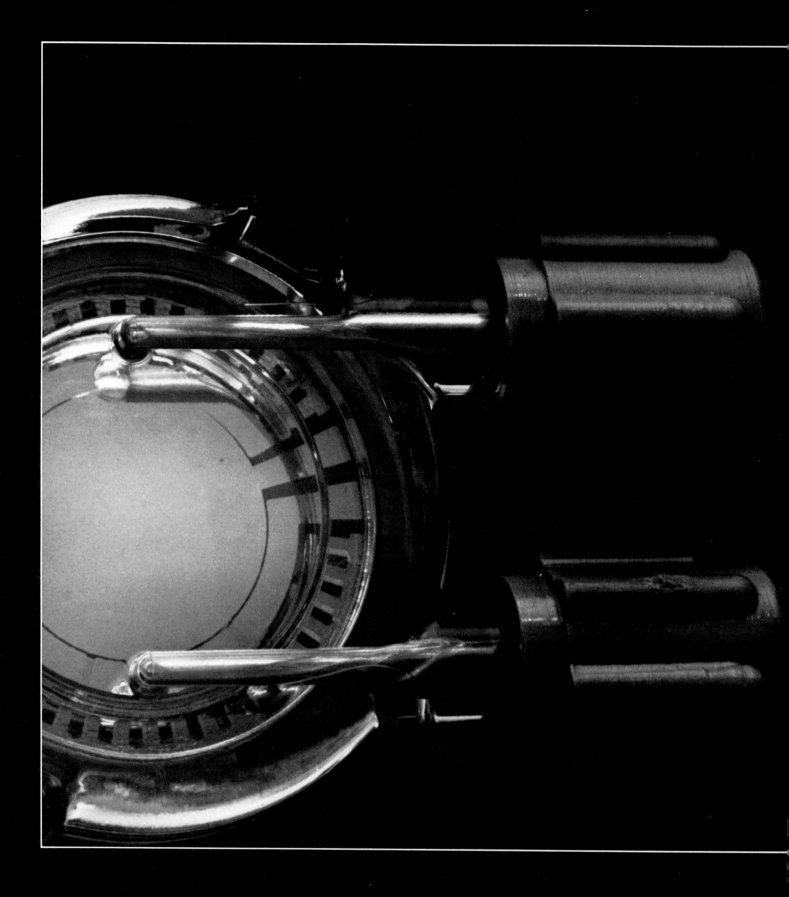

Measuring Hemodynamic Pressure

Hemodynamic monitoring basics

Arterial line

Pulmonary artery line

Left atrial line

Hemodynamic monitoring basics

Hemodynamic monitoring. You do it every time you take a patient's blood pressure with a sphygmomanometer. But how much do you know about *invasive* hemodynamic monitoring?

In this section, you'll learn about all types of invasive hemodynamic monitoring, from peripheral arterial lines to balloon-tipped pulmonary artery lines that thread through the heart's right chambers. But first, you need some background information.

Throughout the next few pages, we'll discuss the pros and cons of hemodynamic monitoring and review the cardiac cycle, so you know exactly what monitoring tells you. In addition, we'll introduce some of the equipment you'll use for any hemodynamic line. And finally, we'll show you how to troubleshoot common hemodynamic monitoring problems.

In other words, we'll cover the basics. Read these pages carefully. Then, when we explain specific monitoring lines, you'll have the background you need.

Hemodynamic monitoring: Pros and cons

Invasive hemodynamic monitoring poses risks for your patient. But for most critically ill patients, the advantages far outweigh the disadvantages. Here are the pros and cons you should know:

Advantages
- Permits accurate, continuous blood pressure readings, even when your patient's in shock and noninvasive methods of pressure monitoring fail
- Reveals subtle changes in your patient's cardiovascular system that are undetectable by noninvasive methods
- Reflects your patient's immediate response to medication, therapy, or stress.

Disadvantages
- Increases the risk of complications for the patient; for example, infection, bleeding, embolism, and tissue or blood vessel damage. In addition, the introduction of a pulmonary artery catheter may cause cardiac arrhythmias
- Requires specialized training to use. Otherwise, you may not recognize (or know how to correct) possible errors or inaccuracies in the monitoring system
- May give you a false sense of security. Remember, monitoring is only one part of complete nursing care.

Reviewing the heart's anatomy

The heart is a hollow, muscular pump that generates hemodynamic pressures with strong, rhythmic contractions. Brush up on its anatomical features by studying the two views of the heart illustrated on the opposite page.

Your patient's heart is just a little larger than his clenched fist. It's shaped something like an inverted pyramid—widest at the top and narrowest at the bottom—and rests in the *mediastinum* (the space between his lungs).But, as you probably know, the heart doesn't lie precisely in the middle of the thoracic cavity. Because of its forward slanting position, more than two-thirds of it lies to the *left* of midline. Its narrow tip (or apex) lies farthest forward, resting on the left side of the diaphragm.

Although we don't show it here, the heart is protected by a baggy, multi-layered sac called the *pericardium*. The slippery pericardial fluid found between two of these layers lubricates the sac as the heart beats.

Study these illustrations to better understand the heart's anatomy. Then, review them as often as necessary when you read these pages on hemodynamic monitoring.

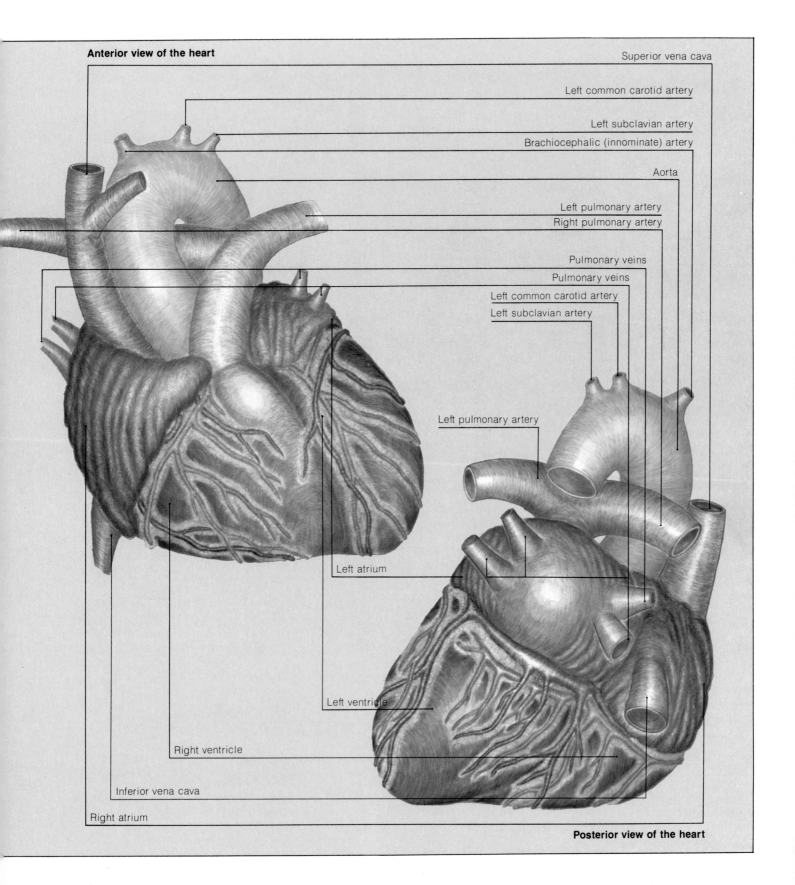

Anterior view of the heart

Superior vena cava

Left common carotid artery

Left subclavian artery

Brachiocephalic (innominate) artery

Aorta

Left pulmonary artery

Right pulmonary artery

Pulmonary veins

Pulmonary veins

Left common carotid artery

Left subclavian artery

Left pulmonary artery

Left atrium

Left ventricle

Right ventricle

Inferior vena cava

Right atrium

Posterior view of the heart

Hemodynamic monitoring basics

Understanding the cardiac cycle

You can't understand the value of hemo-dynamic monitoring without first under-standing the cardiac cycle. Of course, you studied it thor-oughly in nursing school, so you have good background knowledge. Use this page as a review.

As you know, the cardiac cycle has two phases: diastole, when the heart's ventricles fill with blood from the atria; and sys-tole, when the ven-tricles contract and eject the blood. During diastole, the right ventricle fills with venous blood from the su-perior vena cava. During systole, it ejects this blood into the pulmonary artery. Then, the pulmonary artery carries this blood to the lungs, for oxy-genation.

As the right ventri-cle fills with venous blood, the left ven-tricle fills with oxy-genated blood returning from the lungs. During sys-tole, the left ventri-cle ejects this oxygenated blood into the aorta, which distributes it to the rest of the body.

Now, let's take a detailed look at the diastolic phase of the cardiac cycle. To do this, examine the following illustra-tions.

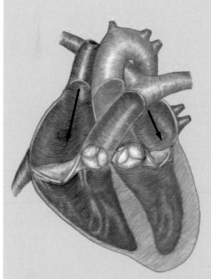

1 At the beginning of the diastolic phase of the cardiac cycle, the following valves are closed: the atrioventricular (mitral and tricuspid) and the semilunar (aortic and pulmonic). The atria begin to fill with blood.

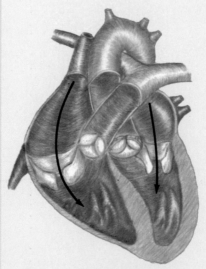

2 As the atria fill, ventricular pressure drops. When it's lower than atrial pressure, the atrioventricular valves open, as shown here. Blood rushes from the atria into the ventricles, causing rapid ventricular filling.

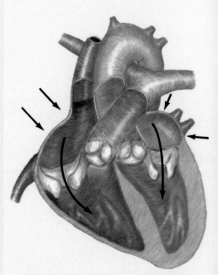

3 As blood continues to fill the ventricles, ventricular pressure rises and atrial pressure drops. Rising ventricular pressure slows blood flow from the atria. Then, as you see here, the atria contract, forcing enough blood into the ventricles to fill them completely.

4 Now that the ventricles are full, let's take a closer look at just the *left* side of the heart. Remember, because this side expels blood to the rest of the body, it works harder than the right side. That's why heart failure usually occurs on the heart's left side before the right.

The amount of blood in the left ventricle at the end of diastole is called *left ventricular end diastolic volume* (LVEDV). The pressure it exerts on the left ventricle's walls is called *left ventricular end diastolic pressure* (LVEDP). The combination of LVEDV and LVEDP is called preload. Preload's affected by many factors, such as blood volume, heart muscle condition, and the blood vessels' ability to constrict and dilate. In many cases, cardiac therapy aims to reduce preload, so the left side of the heart doesn't need to work as hard. Pulmonary artery wedge pressure (PAWP) is a good indicator of preload, because it reflects any pressure changes in the left side of the heart.

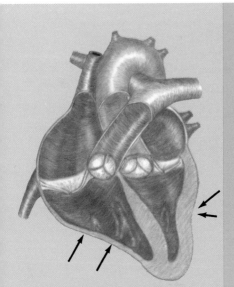

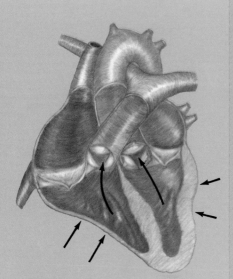

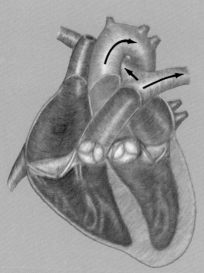

5 Now, consider the systolic phase of the cardiac cycle. After the ventricles have filled completely, the atrioventricular valves close. Since the semilunar valves are also closed, the ventricles are now completely closed chambers.

Next, the ventricles begin contracting, as shown here, increasing intraventricular pressure.

6 When intraventricular pressures exceed aortic and pulmonic pressures, the semilunar valves open. Blood is then ejected from the right ventricle into the pulmonary artery, and from the left ventricle into the aorta. (About 75% of the heart's blood is ejected during this phase.)

7 As the ventricles eject blood, pulmonary artery and aortic pressures rise. When these pressures are greater than ventricular pressures, the semilunar valves close and the cardiac cycle's complete.

8 Once again, let's take a closer look at the left side of the heart. When the left ventricle ejects its blood, it must overcome aortic pressure, or *afterload*. Afterload is estimated by comparing the patient's systemic arterial pressure, his cardiac output, and his pulmonary artery pressure.

The amount of blood remaining in the left ventricle at the end of systole (normally 50 to 60 ml) is called the *left ventricular end systolic volume* (LVESV). Stroke volume (the amount of blood ejected by the left ventricle with each contraction) is the difference between LVEDV and LVESV. You can also calculate stroke volume by dividing cardiac output by heart rate. In a healthy adult, stroke volume is usually about 70 ml.

Cardiac output is the amount of blood ejected per minute by the left ventricle. Calculate cardiac output by multiplying the patient's heart rate with his stroke volume. If your patient has a pulmonary artery (PA) line that includes a thermistor, you can use a special computerized monitor to determine cardiac output directly.

Hemodynamic monitoring basics

How hemodynamic waveforms reflect the cardiac cycle

How does the monitor's oscilloscope or readout strip reflect the cardiac cycle? This chart illustrates how hemodynamic waveforms correspond to EKG waveforms.

Notice how the hemodynamic waveform lags slightly behind the EKG waveform here and on your oscilloscope screen or readout strip. That's because the EKG's electrical signal reaches the monitor slightly before the transducer's signal.

Look at the cardiac cycle phases marked at the top of the page. We've included them here to show you how hemodynamic and EKG waveforms correspond to diastole and systole.

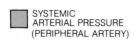 SYSTEMIC ARTERIAL PRESSURE (PERIPHERAL ARTERY)

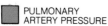 PULMONARY ARTERY PRESSURE

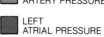 LEFT ATRIAL PRESSURE

CENTRAL VENOUS PRESSURE (RIGHT ATRIUM)

 EKG

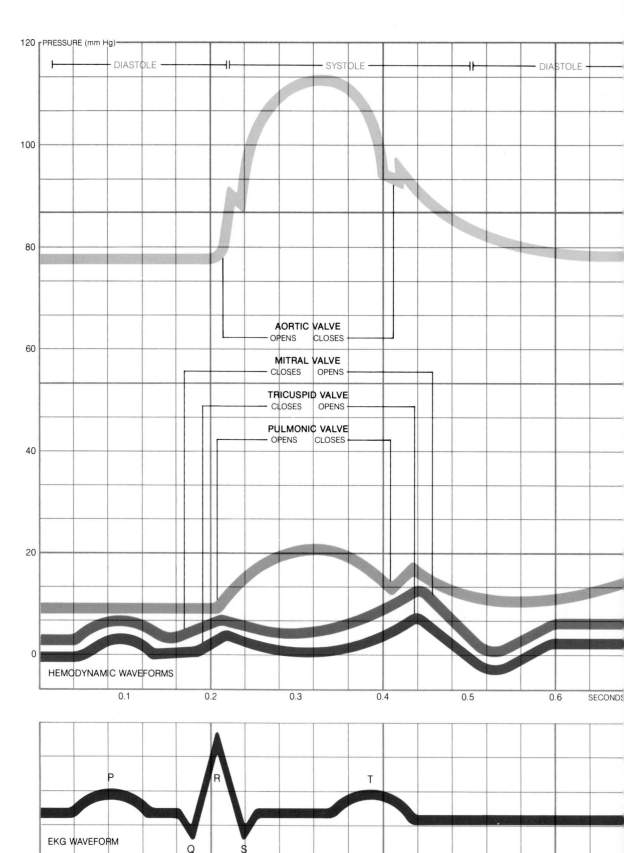

PRESSURE (mm Hg)

DIASTOLE — SYSTOLE — DIASTOLE

AORTIC VALVE
OPENS   CLOSES

MITRAL VALVE
CLOSES   OPENS

TRICUSPID VALVE
CLOSES   OPENS

PULMONIC VALVE
OPENS   CLOSES

HEMODYNAMIC WAVEFORMS

SECONDS

EKG WAVEFORM

Assembling your equipment

When we discuss specific hemodynamic pressure monitoring lines in this PHOTOBOOK, we explain exactly what equipment to gather. But some equipment's indispensable for *any* hemodynamic monitoring line using a transducer. In the following paragraphs, you'll discover what this equipment is and why it's essential:

• *Pressure bag.* Because the blood flow in a patient's arteries and central veins exerts such strong pressure, you must infuse I.V. flush solution under pressure (usually 300 mm Hg). The pressure bag works only on I.V. flush solutions packaged in a bag.

• *I.V. flush solution (either sterile normal saline solution, or 5% dextrose in water).* Most doctors prefer normal saline solution, because it doesn't support bacteria growth as well as 5% dextrose in water does. However, 5% dextrose in water will cause less strain on your patient's heart in case of accidental fluid overload. In addition, 5% dextrose in water is a poor electrical conductor, so it enhances electrical safety during monitoring. *Important:* If a left atrial line's inserted, 5% dextrose in water is the solution of choice.

• *Heparin.* To reduce risk of clotting at catheter tip, inject heparin directly into the flush solution (1 to 2 units heparin per ml of solution).

• *Rigid pressure tubing.* If you use regular I.V. tubing, it will expand under high hemodynamic pressures and distort readings.

• *Continuous flush device.* This helps keep the line patent by maintaining a continuous flow rate of 3 to 4 ml per hour. In addition, it allows safe, fast flushing. (For details on the Sorenson Intraflo™ continuous flush device, see the photostory on the right.

Using a Sorenson Intraflo™ continuous flush device

1 Are you monitoring your patient's hemodynamic pressure? This Sorenson Intraflo continuous flush device allows heparinized solution infused under pressure to flush the line continuously at a rate of 3 to 4 ml per hour. As you know, continuous flushing helps prevent blood clotting; the slow rate reduces the risk of fluid overload. You'll use this device—or one like it—on nearly all hemodynamic lines.

The handy rubber tail attached to the fast flush valve on this device is commonly called the pigtail. This valve lets you routinely fast flush the line to further reduce the risk of blood clotting. Unlike flushing with a syringe (which may force a large clot into the patient's bloodstream), fast flushing is safe. The fast flush valve releases only a small amount of fluid under limited pressure. As a result, ejection of a large clot is unlikely.

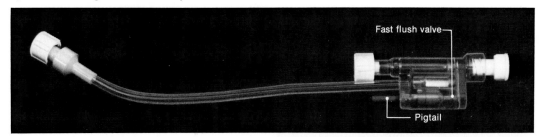

Fast flush valve

Pigtail

2 To fast flush a hemodynamic pressure monitoring line, first make sure the stopcock is turned so it's open from container to patient. Check to determine that the transducer's open to the line, too. Then, pull the pigtail firmly, and release it with a snap. (Snapping the pigtail ensures that the valve closes completely.) Fast flush the line at least once each hour, as well as after withdrawing a blood sample. *Important:* Avoid rapid, repeated flushing, which can cause turbulence and produce air bubbles.

[Inset] As you fast flush the line, watch the I.V. bag's drip chamber. The fluid should flow rapidly for several seconds, then resume its steady, slow flow. If the fluid doesn't flow more rapidly when you fast flush, the catheter may be clotted or may have pulled out of the blood vessel. Locate and correct the problem at once.

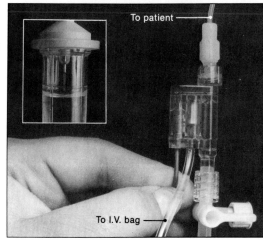

To patient

To I.V. bag

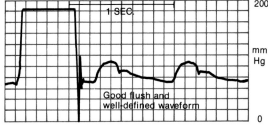

Good flush and well-defined waveform

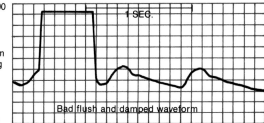

200

mm Hg

0

Bad flush and damped waveform

3 What does the waveform on the monitor look like when you fast flush the line? Compare these two illustrations. When you pull and release the pigtail, the oscilloscope screen or readout strip should show a square waveform that descends to the zero level, like the one on the left. If you get a square waveform that doesn't zero, followed by a damped waveform (like the one on the right), suspect a partial occlusion in the line or catheter. Locate and correct the problem. (For troubleshooting tips on how to do this, see the chart on page 78.)

After flushing the line, examine the I.V. bag's drip chamber to check the drip rate. The rate should be 3 to 4 ml per hour. If the rate's faster, you may have a stuck fast flush valve, or a loose connection in the line. Tighten all connections. Then, try flushing the line again, remembering to release the pigtail with a snap. If the flow rate doesn't slow immediately, replace the continuous flush device. *Note:* The Sorenson Intraflo is the most commonly used continuous flush device. However, other types are available; for example, the Gould Critiflo™ device. For details, see pages 88 and 89.

Hemodynamic monitoring basics

Troubleshooting a damped waveform

You probably know what damped waveforms look like. Unlike sharply defined waveforms, damped waveforms, which lack definition, are smooth and wavy in appearance, and abnormally low. (You'll see an example of one at the bottom of page 42.) But do you know how to correct damped waveforms, as well as how to prevent them from occurring? Read this chart to find out.

Possible cause	Nursing action	Prevention
Air bubbles somewhere in line; for example, tubing, transducer dome, or stopcocks	• Check stopcocks and make sure they're positioned correctly. • Check the line for leaks. Replace the tubing and stopcocks, if necessary. • Check for loose connections, especially dome connections, and tighten them, if necessary. • Flush out air through an open stopcock port.	• Flush all air from line when setting up equipment. • Avoid rapid, repeated pulling of the pigtail on the fast flush valve. This causes turbulence in the flushing solution, which, in turn, produces air bubbles.
Blood clot in catheter or stopcock	• Pull the pigtail on the fast flush valve to flush the catheter, *but do not attempt this on a left atrial line*. • Try to aspirate the clotted blood with a syringe. Again, *do not* attempt this on a left atrial line. *Important:* Never *flush* any hemodynamic line with a syringe. You may cause an embolus. • If the catheter remains clotted, notify the doctor and prepare to replace the line.	• Maintain adequate flow rate of heparinized flush solution (3 to 4 ml per hour). • Use the fast flush valve to flush the catheter after drawing blood samples.
Arterial catheter has been pulled out of blood vessel or is pressed against vessel wall	• Attempt to aspirate blood to confirm proper placement in vessel. (*Do not* attempt this on a left atrial line.) • If you can't aspirate blood, notify doctor and prepare to replace the line. *Note:* Bloody drainage at the insertion site may indicate catheter displacement. Notify the doctor at once.	• Tape the catheter securely. • Stabilize the insertion site with a splint.
Pulmonary artery (PA) catheter pressed or wedged against blood vessel wall	• Deflate balloon on PA catheter completely. • Ask patient to cough. This may jolt the catheter free. • Fast flush the catheter. This also may jolt it free. • Notify the doctor, so he can reposition the catheter, if necessary. • Prepare the patient for a chest X-ray to confirm correct catheter placement.	• Make sure the catheter is securely sutured and taped. • Observe PA waveforms closely. • Make sure the balloon's *completely* deflated after each use.
Regular I.V. tubing used as part of the setup	• Replace I.V. tubing with rigid pressure tubing.	• Always use rigid pressure tubing for hemodynamic pressure monitoring. Regular I.V. tubing expands under pressure, causing damped waveforms.
Transducer not balanced properly	• Check transducer cable for occlusion or compression. • Level the transducer's balancing port with the patient's right atrium, and balance the transducer to atmospheric pressure. • Recalibrate the monitor with the transducer. (For details on balancing and calibrating, see pages 16 to 18.)	• Keep transducer cable off the floor so it isn't damaged. • Reposition the transducer whenever the patient's position changes. Remember, its balancing port must always be level with the patient's right atrium. • Rebalance and recalibrate equipment if the room temperature changes significantly. • Rebalance and recalibrate equipment at least once every 8 hours. ⊟ *Nursing tip:* When using a standard-sized transducer, avoid putting more than two or three drops of sterile water between the transducer and the dome. Too much fluid can damp the waveform.
Blood backup in line	• Check stopcock positions and make sure they're correct. • Check for loose connections and tighten them, if necessary. • Use the fast flush valve to flush blood from catheter. *Do not* attempt this on a left atrial line. • Replace dome if blood backs up into it.	• Maintain 300 mm Hg of pressure in the pressure bag at all times.

Troubleshooting other common hemodynamic pressure monitoring problems

On the preceding pages, you learned how to troubleshoot a damped waveform. Read this chart to learn about other common hemodynamic monitoring problems. You'll see what may cause them, as well as how to deal with them.

Problem	Possible causes	Nursing action
No waveform	• Power supply off. • Oscilloscope's pressure range set too low. • Loose connection in line • Transducer's stopcock off to patient. • Catheter's occluded or out of blood vessel.	• Check power supply. • Reset oscilloscope's pressure range higher, if necessary. Then, rebalance and recalibrate the equipment. • Tighten any loose connections, and position stopcocks correctly. • Use fast flush valve to flush line, but *do not* attempt this on a left atrial line. • Try to aspirate blood from the catheter, but do not attempt this on a left atrial line. If the line still won't flush, notify the doctor and prepare to replace the line.
Drifting waveforms	• Monitor and transducer not warmed up properly. • Monitor's electrical cable compressed. • Temperature change in room air or I.V. flush solution	• Allow monitor and transducer to warm up 10 to 15 minutes. • Place monitor's cable where it can't be stepped on or compressed. • Remember to routinely rebalance and recalibrate 30 minutes after setting up the equipment. This gives the I.V. fluid sufficient time to warm to room temperature.
Line won't flush	• Stopcocks positioned incorrectly. • Inadequate pressure from pressure bag • Kink in pressure tubing or blood clot in catheter	• Check stopcocks to make sure they're positioned correctly. • Check pressure bag to make sure pressure reads 300 mm Hg. • Check pressure tubing for kinks. • Try aspirating blood clot with a syringe, but *do not* attempt this on a left atrial line. • If the line still won't flush, notify the doctor and prepare to replace the line. *Important:* Never use a syringe to *flush* any hemodynamic line.
Artifact (waveform interference)	• Patient movement • Electrical interference • Catheter fling (tip of pulmonary artery catheter moving rapidly in large blood vessel or heart chamber)	• Wait until the patient's quiet before taking a reading. • Make sure electrical equipment's connected and grounded correctly. • Notify doctor of catheter fling. He may try to reposition the catheter.
False high readings	• Transducer's balancing port positioned below the patient's right atrium • Transducer unbalanced • Flush solution flow rate too fast • Catheter fling	• Position the transducer's balancing port level with the patient's right atrium. • Check transducer's cable, and make sure it's not kinked or occluded. • Rebalance and recalibrate the equipment. • Check flow rate of flush solution. Maintain it at 3 to 4 ml per hour. • Notify doctor of catheter fling. He may try to reposition the catheter.
False low readings	• Transducer's balancing port positioned above the patient's right atrium. • Loose connection in line	• Position the transducer's balancing port level with the patient's right atrium. • Check all connections and tighten them, if necessary.

Arterial line

Your patient needs continuous blood pressure readings, so the doctor's inserted an arterial catheter and connected it to a monitor. Why doesn't he just order repeated blood pressure cuff readings instead?

The answer's easy: blood pressure cuff readings aren't always accurate, especially when the patient's hypotensive. And if your patient's critically ill, accuracy's essential.

Arterial line blood pressure monitoring, however, is highly reliable. After the line's in place, you can check the patient's blood pressure frequently and efficiently without disturbing him. What's more, you can draw frequent blood samples through the line without repeated venipunctures. (For details on drawing arterial blood samples, see the *Nursing80* PHOTOBOOK *Providing Respiratory Care.*)

But suppose your patient isn't critically ill. In that case, the doctor may want you to monitor the patient's arterial blood pressure with a noninvasive ultrasound monitoring system instead. In the following pages, you'll see how to use one.

No matter which method you use to monitor your patient's blood pressure, your role is challenging. Make sure you can meet that challenge by reading these pages.

Choosing an arterial catheter site

When the doctor performs an arterial catheter insertion on your patient, he'll probably choose either a radial or a brachial artery. But if these arteries are unavailable because of burns or other injuries to the patient's arms, he may choose a femoral or a dorsalis pedis artery. This chart describes the pros and cons of each.

BRACHIAL ARTERY

Advantages
• Larger than radial artery and easily located
• Site readily observed and maintained
• Bleeding can usually be prevented or controlled by direct pressure.
• Pressure readings may be more accurate than those taken from the radial artery, since the site's closer to the heart.

Disadvantages
• Risk of damage to median nerves during catheter insertion.
• Risk of tissue damage if artery occludes, because patient will lack adequate collateral circulation to the lower arm.
• Patient's elbow must be splinted to stabilize the catheter, causing joint stiffness.
• Thrombosis may occur if artery's small (in children and small women) or if patient has low cardiac output.

RADIAL ARTERY

Advantages
• Easily located
• Ulnar artery provides good collateral circulation to hand.
• Site readily observed and maintained
• Anatomically stable; radius acts as natural splint.

Disadvantages
• Small lumen in vessel; catheter insertion may be difficult and painful.
• Pressure readings may be inaccurately high, because site is so far from heart.

FEMORAL ARTERY

Advantages
• Large lumen in vessel; may be the easiest artery to locate and puncture in an emergency
• Anatomically stable; femur acts as natural splint

Disadvantages
• Risk of damage to nearby femoral vein and major nerves during catheter insertion
• High risk of thrombosis
• Risk of tissue damage if artery occludes, because of limited collateral circulation
• Difficult to secure catheter
• Difficult to bandage insertion site and keep it clean
• Difficult to prevent and control bleeding

DORSALIS PEDIS ARTERY

Advantages
• May be used if other sites are unavailable because of burns or other injuries

Disadvantages
• High risk of thrombosis
• Produces false high blood pressure readings, because site is so far from heart.

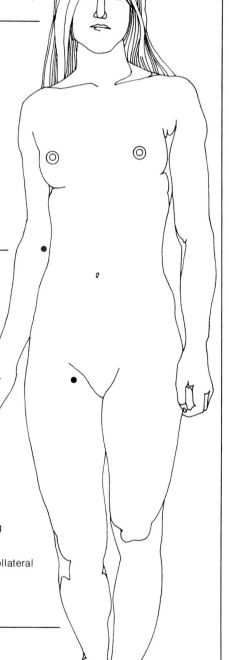

Selecting an arterial line catheter

When the doctor wants to insert an arterial line catheter, what kind will he choose? Most likely, he'll select an over-the-needle catheter (ONC), which is inserted percutaneously. (However, if the patient's condition requires it, the doctor may choose a cutdown catheter instead.)

If the doctor chooses an ONC for your patient, expect it to be:
• made of rigid, nontoxic plastic. Flexible plastic distorts the pressure reading.
• about 2" long. This length is long enough to rest securely in the artery, but short enough to minimize distortion of the pressure reading.
• between 14 and 18 gauge in diameter, for an adult. For a child, use the largest gauge possible, depending on his size. A large catheter decreases the risk of clotting.
• radiopaque, for easy location by X-ray in case of catheter migration or catheter embolism.

PATIENT PREPARATION

Preparing your patient

If your patient needs an arterial line, make sure you've prepared him properly before the doctor begins the insertion. Here's how:
• Explain the procedure to your patient. Tell him that the doctor will give him a local anesthetic to minimize discomfort. Then, take time to answer his questions completely. Remember, catheter insertion is easier if your patient's relaxed.
• Find out if your patient's allergic to the povodine-iodine skin prep or the local anesthetic. If he's allergic to either, tell the doctor.
• If the doctor's chosen the radial artery for the insertion site, check your patient's ulnar and radial artery circulation using the Allen's test (see the next photostory).
• Document your patient's pulse distal to the chosen insertion site. If his pulse weakens later while the arterial catheter's in place, suspect inadequate blood circulation.
• Position your patient so he's comfortable. Make sure the insertion site's level and easily accessible.
• Protect your patient's bed linens by placing a bedsaver pad under the insertion site. Cover the bedsaver pad with a sterile towel.

How to do the Allen's test

Before the doctor inserts an arterial line in one of your patient's radial arteries, you must perform the Allen's test to assess the blood supply to your patient's hand. Why? Because if the radial artery's blocked by a blood clot (a frequent complication of arterial lines), the ulnar artery alone must supply blood to the hand. The Allen's test is a simple, reliable procedure that quickly tells you how well both arteries function. Just follow these steps:

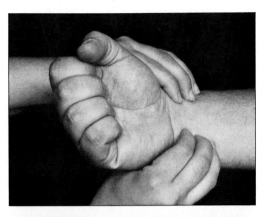

1 With your fingers, compress both the ulnar and radial arteries at your patient's wrist for about 1 minute. Ask your patient to clench and unclench his fist to encourage his palm to blanch.
🕭 *Nursing tip:* Suppose your patient's unconscious or unable to clench his fist for some other reason. You can encourage his palm to blanch by occluding both arteries, elevating his hand, and massaging his palm.

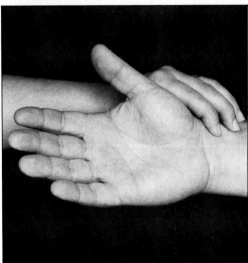

2 Release the pressure on the ulnar artery, and ask the patient to open his hand. If the ulnar artery's functioning well, his palm will turn pink in about 5 seconds, even though the radial artery's still occluded. But if blood return is slow and his fingers begin to contract, blood supply from the radial artery may not be adequate. In that case, try the Allen's test on his other wrist; you may get better results. *Note:* Slow blood return doesn't always indicate arterial occlusion. It may indicate poor cardiac output or poor capillary refill, resulting from shock.

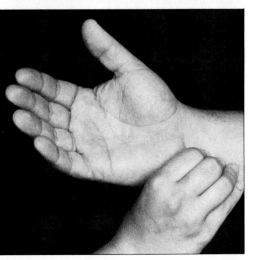

3 Is the ulnar artery's blood return OK? Then repeat the procedure, this time releasing just the radial artery. Remember, both arteries must function well to assure adequate blood supply to the hand while an arterial line's in place. If radial blood return is slow, perform the test on your patient's other wrist.

If blood return is slow in either artery on both wrists, tell the doctor. He may choose another site.

Arterial line

How to set up equipment for arterial blood pressure monitoring

1 *Have you prepared the patient properly, following the guidelines on the preceding page? If so, you're ready to set up the equipment needed for arterial blood pressure monitoring. On the following pages, we'll show you how. (In practice, the procedure may differ slightly, depending on your hospital's equipment and policy.)* First, obtain a monitor, I.V. pole, sphygmomanometer, leveling arm, and transducer holder. Then, wash your hands and gather the equipment shown here: pressure bag, 500 ml bag normal saline solution, label, transducer, transducer dome, 3 cc syringe and 1½" needle, syringe (with needle) filled with 1,000 units heparin, alcohol swab, two-way stopcock, two three-

way stopcocks, male adapter plug, micro-drip I.V. pressure tubing, 4' pressure tubing, 6" pressure tubing, continuous flush device, and sterile water. (If the doctor wants you to apply a dressing, you'll need antimicrobial ointment, an adhesive bandage strip, a splint, and 2" wide adhesive tape.) Maintain aseptic technique throughout the procedure.

Turn on the monitor and plug in the transducer, so they can warm up while you work. *Note:* Replace vented stopcock caps with closed ones before you begin.

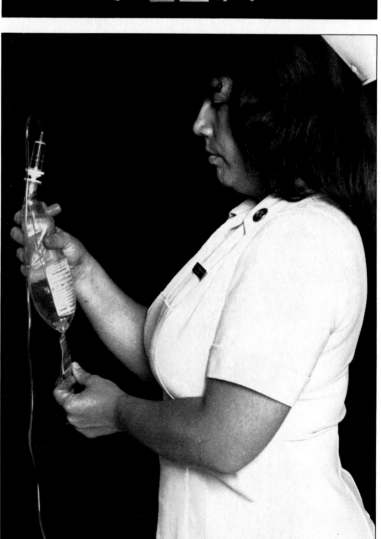

2 Label the I.V. saline solution bag with the patient's name, the time and date, and your initials. In addition, include the amount of heparin you'll inject into the I.V. bag. Then, spike and invert the bag. Squeeze out all the air through the drip chamber, as shown here. Expelling the air reduces the risk of later forcing an air bubble into the patient's artery. Close the line's flow clamp. Then, hang the bag on the I.V. pole.

3 Inject the heparin into the I.V. bag, as shown in the photo below. Heparin prevents clotting in the line. Most hospitals use 1 or 2 units of heparin per ml saline solution.

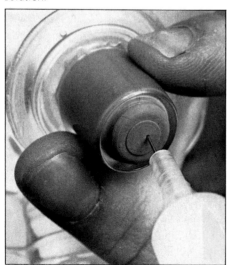

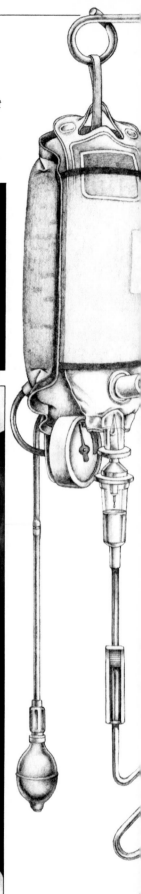

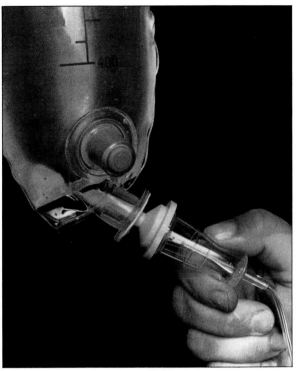

4 Squeeze the drip chamber until it's half full. To avoid causing turbulence in the saline solution, squeeze the drip chamber slowly and rhythmically.

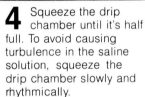 *Nursing tip:* As you squeeze, tilt the drip chamber sideways. This helps prevent air bubbles from forming as the drip chamber fills.

Now, open the line's flow clamp, and prime the tubing until all air bubbles are flushed from the tubing. Close the clamp. *Important:* Since you'll be infusing the solution under pressure, flushing air bubbles from the tubing is especially important. Otherwise, you may later force air into the patient's bloodstream, causing an embolism. Always take care to eliminate air bubbles at every step of the procedure, as well as when you change any part of the equipment.

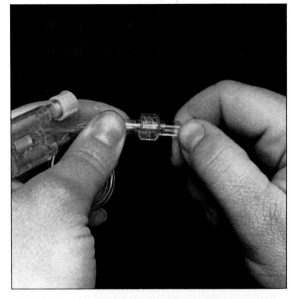

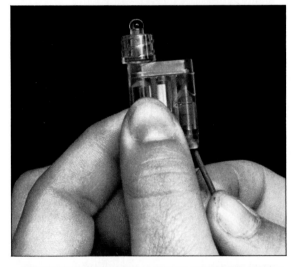

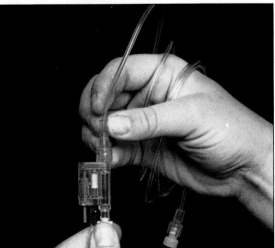

5 Next, attach a continuous flush device to the line, and screw it on *tightly.*

Important: Make sure all connections are secure. A disconnection in an arterial line can cause serious—possibly fatal—bleeding.

6 To flush the air from the continuous flush device, uncap the Luer-Lok™ port and hold it upright, as shown here. This vertical position encourages air bubbles to rise and escape. Open the flow clamp, and pull the pigtail on the continuous flush device until the saline solution runs out the Luer-Lok port. Release the pigtail.

7 Next, attach the 4' pressure tubing to the Luer-Lok port, as shown here.

Arterial line

How to set up equipment for arterial blood pressure monitoring continued

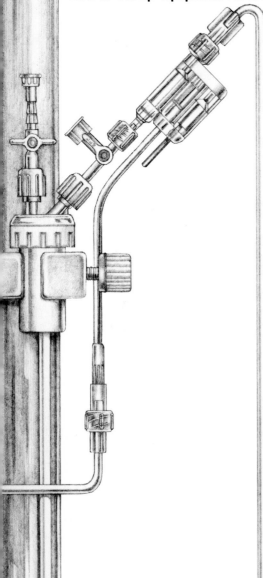

8 Uncap the *Luer-Tip* port and hold it upright. (Notice that this port is a little larger than the Luer-Lok port, so air escapes from it more easily.) As shown here, pull the pigtail until saline solution runs out the port. Hold the pigtail taut until all air bubbles are expelled. Then, cap the Luer-Tip port.

Nursing tip: Expel stubborn air bubbles by flicking the continuous flush device with your finger. When the air bubbles rise to the top, pull the pigtail to flush them out.

9 Uncap the 4' pressure tubing, and pull the pigtail to flush it, also.

10 When the 4' pressure tubing has been completely flushed, attach a three-way stopcock to the end of it. For easy reference, we'll call this Stopcock #1.

11 Attach the 6" pressure tubing to Stopcock #1, as shown here.

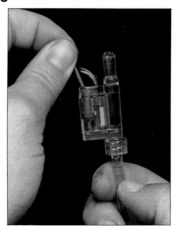

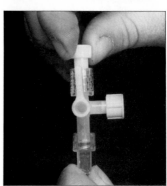

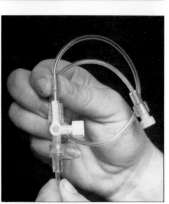

12 Turn Stopcock #1 off to the middle port, and uncap the 6" pressure tubing. Flush the 6" pressure tubing by pulling the pigtail. (Remember to hold the end of the tubing upright, so air bubbles rise to the top.) Examine the tubing closely to make sure all the air's expelled. When you're sure it is, cap the end of the line.

13 Turn Stopcock #1 off to the 6" pressure tubing. Now the line's open between the bag and the stopcock's middle port. Remove the cap from the middle port, and pull the pigtail until saline solution runs out the port and all the air's expelled. Remember to hold the port upright, so the air can rise.

14 When you're sure the air's out, cap the port with a male adapter plug (injection nipple). *Remember:* Tighten all connections.

15 Uncap the Luer-Tip port of the continuous flush device, and attach a second stopcock (Stopcock #2). Although some nurses don't use a stopcock at this juncture, we recommend it. It permits you to isolate the transducer from the line.

16 Turn Stopcock #2 off to its lateral port. Hold the middle port upright and uncap it. Pull the pigtail to flush the middle port, as shown here. When all the air's expelled, cap the port.

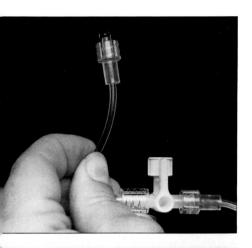

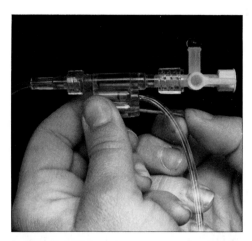

17 Turn Stopcock #2 off to its middle port, and follow the same procedure to flush its lateral port. Remember to hold the lateral port upright, as the nurse is doing here.

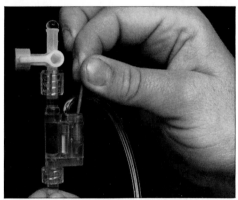

18 Screw one arm of the transducer dome onto the lateral port of Stopcock #2. This leaves the other arm of the dome free for balancing the transducer to atmospheric pressure.

The holder made for this particular transducer allows you to mount the transducer at an angle, so the balancing arm's upright and level. But if the dome you're using has a side arm and an upright arm, leave the *upright* arm free for balancing.

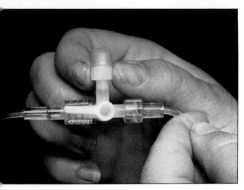

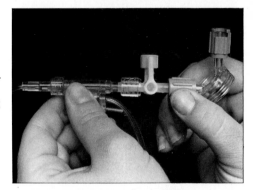

19 Next, place a two-way stopcock (Stopcock #3) on the other arm of the transducer dome. Open the line to the top port. (Remember, the handle position of a two-way stopcock points to an *open* line, not a closed line.)

Hold Stopcock #3 vertically, and remove the cap from its top port. Then, pull the pigtail, as shown, and flush the dome with saline solution. The air will escape through the top port of Stopcock #3. When the dome and Stopcock #3 are free of air, cap Stopcock #3. (If you use a three-way stopcock, make sure you flush all its ports.)

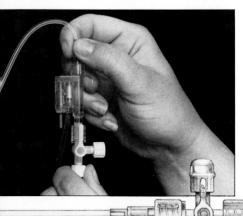

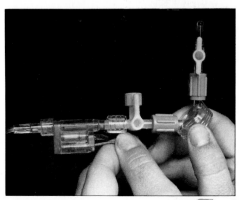

Arterial line

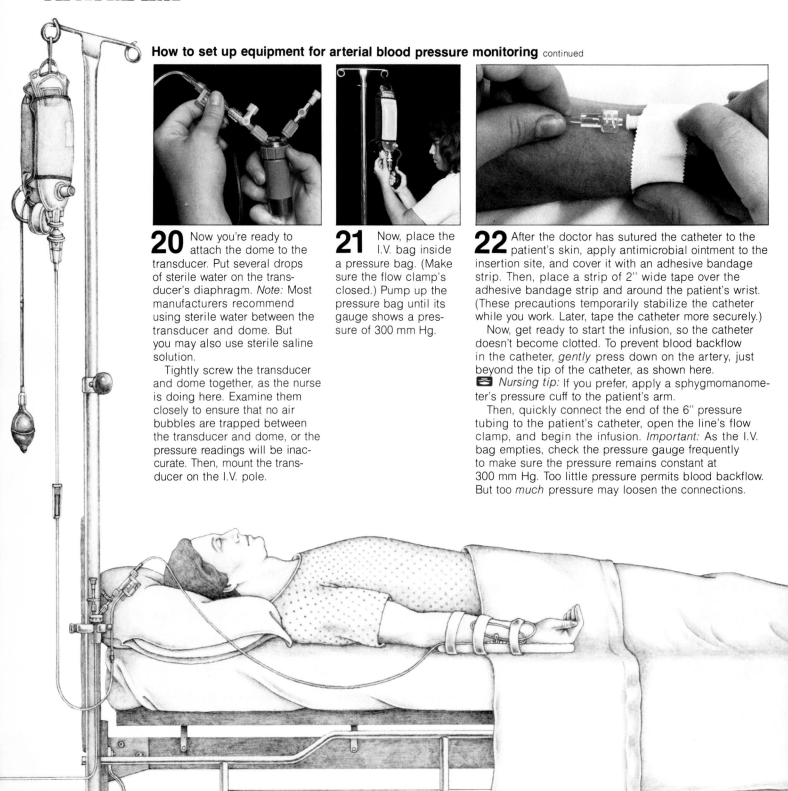

How to set up equipment for arterial blood pressure monitoring continued

20 Now you're ready to attach the dome to the transducer. Put several drops of sterile water on the transducer's diaphragm. *Note:* Most manufacturers recommend using sterile water between the transducer and dome. But you may also use sterile saline solution.

Tightly screw the transducer and dome together, as the nurse is doing here. Examine them closely to ensure that no air bubbles are trapped between the transducer and dome, or the pressure readings will be inaccurate. Then, mount the transducer on the I.V. pole.

21 Now, place the I.V. bag inside a pressure bag. (Make sure the flow clamp's closed.) Pump up the pressure bag until its gauge shows a pressure of 300 mm Hg.

22 After the doctor has sutured the catheter to the patient's skin, apply antimicrobial ointment to the insertion site, and cover it with an adhesive bandage strip. Then, place a strip of 2" wide tape over the adhesive bandage strip and around the patient's wrist. (These precautions temporarily stabilize the catheter while you work. Later, tape the catheter more securely.)

Now, get ready to start the infusion, so the catheter doesn't become clotted. To prevent blood backflow in the catheter, *gently* press down on the artery, just beyond the tip of the catheter, as shown here.

🖀 *Nursing tip:* If you prefer, apply a sphygmomanometer's pressure cuff to the patient's arm.

Then, quickly connect the end of the 6" pressure tubing to the patient's catheter, open the line's flow clamp, and begin the infusion. *Important:* As the I.V. bag empties, check the pressure gauge frequently to make sure the pressure remains constant at 300 mm Hg. Too little pressure permits blood backflow. But too *much* pressure may loosen the connections.

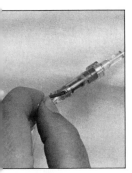

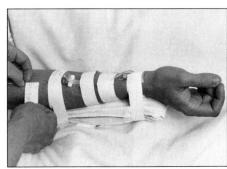

23 Turn the two-way stopcock (Stopcock #3) so it's off to its top port. Then, gently pull the pigtail to flush the line. As you do, watch the drip chamber. If the solution flows steadily and rapidly, the catheter's patent and properly positioned in the patient's artery. Release the pigtail. The drip rate should flow at 3 to 4 ml per hour.

24 When the infusion's flowing properly, finish stabilizing the catheter. Don't neglect this important step; it'll help prevent complications, like arterial spasm or thrombosis.

Here's how: Securely tape the catheter, Stopcock #1, and the 6" pressure tubing to your patient's skin. Loop the 6" pressure tubing to minimize strain on the catheter. Then, if the catheter's inserted in the radial artery, as it is here, apply a short splint (armboard) to your patient's arm to protect it. Label the dressing. *Important:* Leave the stopcock and all connections exposed and accessible, so you can examine them easily.

Finally, label the tubing as an arterial line, as the nurse is doing here. This way, no one will mistake it for an I.V. line.

25 Is the patient's arterial catheter secure? If so, you're ready to balance the transducer. Begin by making sure the patient's flat on his back. Next, locate his right atrium, along the midaxillary line at his fourth intercostal space. Mark the spot with tape.

Then, position the transducer's balancing port (the top port of Stopcock #3) so it's level with the patient's right atrium. Use the leveling arm to do this, or improvise a leveling arm by taping a small medication vial to a yardstick, as the nurse has done here. When the bubble in the vial centers, you know the arm is level.

Why is leveling so important? Because for each inch (2.5 cm) of difference between the balancing port and the right atrium, the pressure reading varies 2 mm Hg. For this reason, you must readjust the level of the balancing port if the patient's position changes.

When the transducer's positioned properly, balance it to atmospheric pressure, and calibrate it with the monitor. (For guidelines on balancing and calibrating, see pages 15 to 18.)

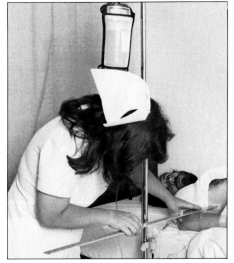

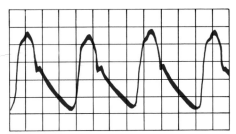

26 After you've finished balancing and calibrating, open the line between the patient and the monitor, and begin monitoring your patient's arterial blood pressure. Look at the waveform on the oscilloscope screen or readout strip. It should be well defined, with a visible dicrotic notch, like the one shown here. If it isn't, try the troubleshooting tips on pages 78 and 79. *Note:* If the catheter's placed in the dorsalis pedis, the dicrotic notch won't be visible on the waveform.

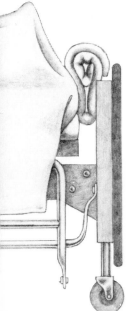

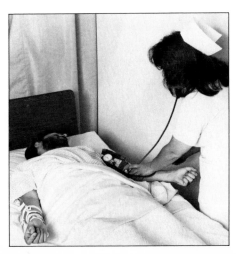

27 Check your patient's blood pressure with a sphygmomanometer to help verify the accuracy of the monitor's pressure reading. When you do, apply the cuff to the arm without the catheter.

Keep in mind that the monitor's blood pressure reading will probably show a higher systole and a lower diastole than your cuff blood pressure reading. Document both readings in your nurses' notes.

Finally, document the entire procedure on your patient's chart and in your nurses' notes. Include this information: insertion site; type and gauge of catheter; doctor's name; I.V. solution's composition (including how much heparin you added), flow rate, and pressure; patient's tolerance of the procedure; patient's pulse (before and after the procedure); color, warmth, and sensation in the area distal to the insertion site; date and time of procedure; and your name.

Double-check all connections to make sure they're secure. At least once an hour, be sure to check the pulse, color, sensation, and mobility of your patient's hand or foot to ensure adequate circulation. In addition, maintain catheter patency by fast flushing the catheter once each hour and whenever you draw a blood sample.

Arterial line

Using a Gould Disposable Critiflo™ Diaphragm Dome

1 *In the previous photostory, you learned how to set up a hemodynamic monitoring line, using a Sorenson Intraflo™ continuous flush device. Here's an alternative to the Intraflo.*

This disposable Critiflo Diaphragm Dome, made by Gould, Inc., operates as a continuous flush device, as well as a transducer dome. Because it eliminates the need for a separate continuous flush device, this dome lets you set up the equipment faster. However, you can use it only with a special transducer made by Gould.

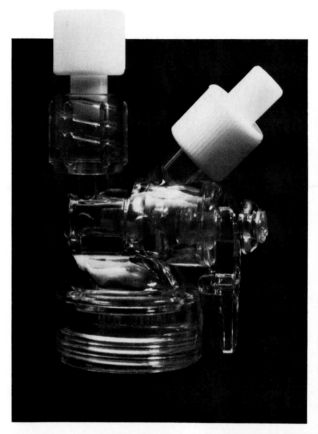

2 Place one or two drops of sterile water on the transducer diaphragm, and attach the dome firmly to the transducer.

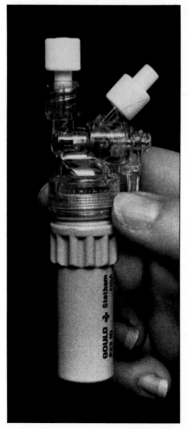

3 Spike the I.V. saline solution bag. Then, prime and flush the tubing, as before. Close the flow clamp. Remove the dome's protective caps, and attach the tubing to the dome's sidearm, as shown here.

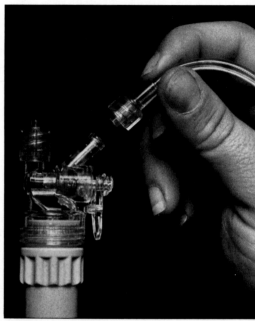

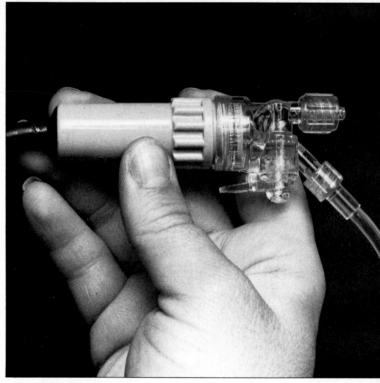

4 Hold the dome like this. Then, open the flow clamp, and let the dome's back chamber fill with fluid. *Don't* press the flush lever yet.

5 When the back chamber's completely filled, hold the dome upright. Then, press the flush lever, and let the dome completely fill with saline solution. Gently tap the dome to expel any air bubbles through the dome's upright arm.

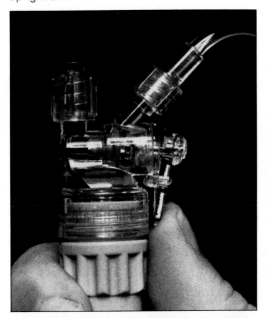

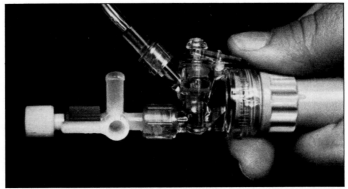

7 Next, attach a protective cap to the airtight cap. Then, hold the middle port upright and remove its cap. Turn the stopcock handle so the line's open to the middle port. Press the lever, as shown here, and flush the middle port.

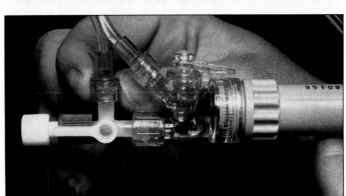

8 Attach the patient's line to the middle port of the stopcock.

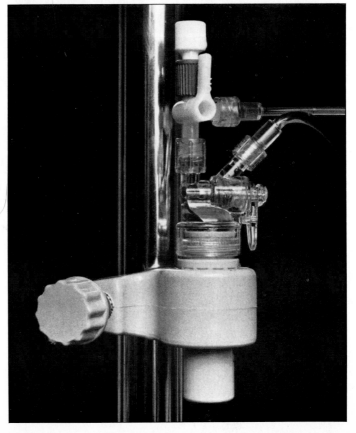

9 Finally, mount the transducer and dome on an I.V. pole, as shown here. Now you're ready to balance the transducer, using the same procedure beginning on page 15.

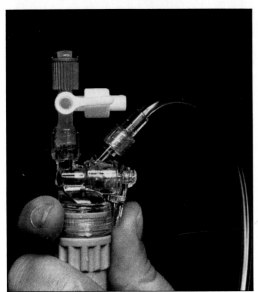

6 Next, attach a three-way stopcock to the dome's upright arm. Turn the stopcock handle so the line's open between the dome and the stopcock's lateral port. Then, press the flush lever, and expel any air bubbles through the lateral port.

The protective cap on this stopcock port isn't airtight; it only guards against touch contamination. The meniscus rising out of its top indicates that the air's been expelled properly.

Arterial line

How to apply a pressure bandage

1 *Let's suppose you've just removed an arterial line. First, apply direct pressure to the site for 5 minutes, if it's a radial site; for 7 minutes, if it's a brachial site; and 10 minutes, if it's a femoral site. Then, as an added precaution, apply a pressure bandage. For this procedure, you'll need 2" wide tape, a 4" x 4" sterile gauze pad, and antimicrobial ointment. Here's how to apply a pressure bandage to a radial site.*

First, cut a piece of 2" tape that's slightly longer than necessary to encircle your patient's wrist. Stick the tape to a handy surface. Apply antimicrobial ointment to the insertion site. Then, fold the 4" x 4" sterile gauze pad once or twice, and press it firmly over the site.

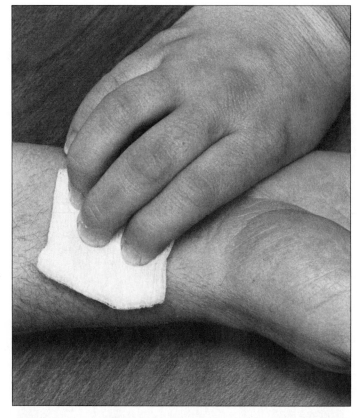

2 Next, firmly wrap the tape around your patient's wrist, pressing down on the gauze pad as you wrap. Let the tape overlap, so it holds the bandage in place.

Important: Never wrap the tape so tightly that it restricts circulation. While the pressure bandage is in place, check your patient's hand frequently for color, pulse, and sensation. At the first sign that the bandage is too tight, loosen it. Or remove it entirely and apply another.

After 1 hour, remove the pressure bandage, and replace it with an adhesive bandage strip.

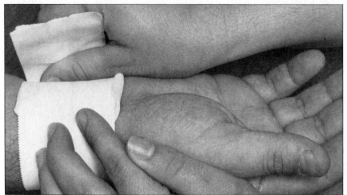

Using an ultrasonic blood pressure monitor

1 *In the following photostory, you'll see how to set up a Roche Arteriosonde® ultrasonic monitor. At preset intervals, this monitor will automatically inflate a pressure cuff you've placed around the patient's arm, take her blood pressure reading, and deflate the cuff. In addition, it'll sound an alarm if your patient's systolic blood pressure reaches a preset high or low level.*

First, gather the equipment shown in this photo: an ultrasonic monitor, transducer, transducer cable, ultrasonic jelly, and the special blood pressure cuff made for this monitor.

2 Explain the procedure to the patient and answer her questions. Then, take her blood pressure with a sphygmomanometer, and record it in your nurses' notes.

Ultrasonic blood pressure monitoring: Advantages and disadvantages

If your patient needs frequent blood pressure monitoring, but doesn't have an arterial catheter in place, you may use a noninvasive ultrasonic monitoring system like the one featured in the following photostory. In the past, ultrasonic monitoring was available only for infants. But now, it's available for adults, too. Here are its advantages and disadvantages.

Advantages
- Noninvasive, so doesn't expose patient to complications like infection and thrombosis
- More accurate than sphygmomanometer pressure cuff monitoring, because the ultrasonic transducer amplifies blood flow sounds

Disadvantages
- Less accurate than an arterial line
- Can't measure blood pressure continuously, like an arterial line, because the cuff pressure needed for this method impairs circulation
- Can't detect extremely low systolic pressures

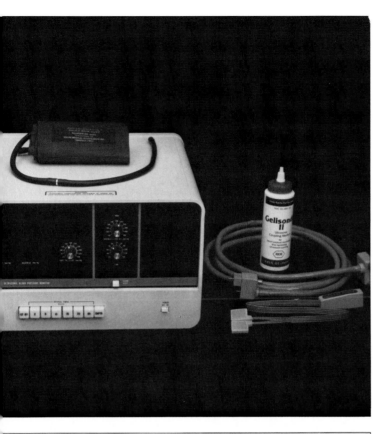

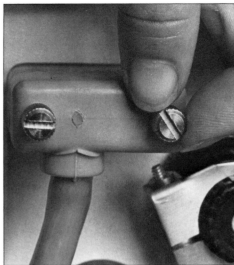

3 Attach the transducer cable to the back of the monitor, as shown here.

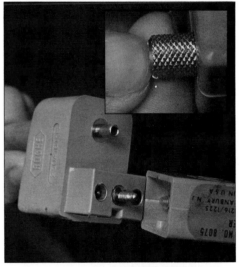

4 Next, fit the transducer onto the *triple* prongs of the cable's plug, as shown here.
[Inset] To secure the transducer, tighten the bottom screw on the back of the cable's plug.

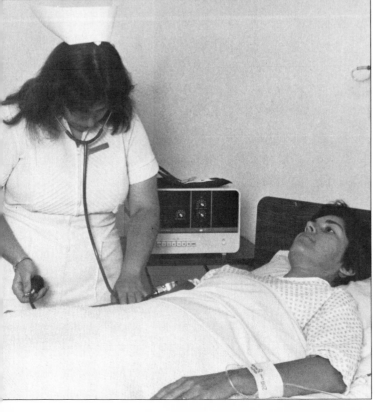

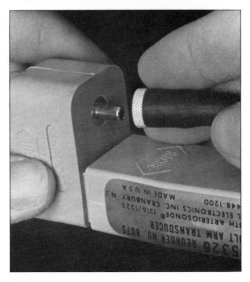

5 Now, locate the *single* prong on the transducer cable's plug. Fit the cable of the blood pressure cuff onto it.

Arterial line

Using an ultrasonic blood pressure monitor continued

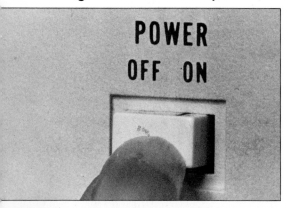

6 Press the POWER button on the front of the monitor to turn it on.

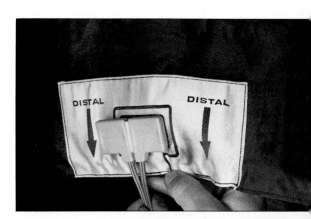

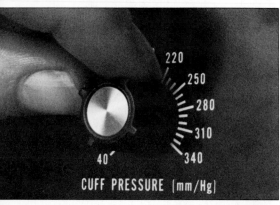

7 Now you're ready to set the monitor. Set the CUFF PRESSURE knob to a pressure that's 30 mm Hg above the patient's *systolic* pressure. (For this you'll use the systolic pressure you measured and recorded when you were explaining the procedure to the patient.) *Important:* As you work, keep in mind that all the settings on this monitor are based on *systolic* pressures, not diastolic pressures.

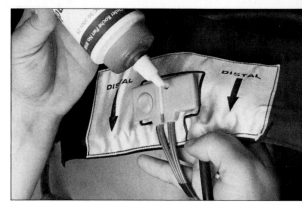

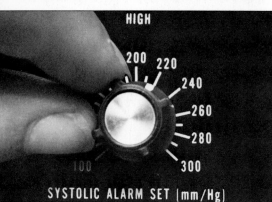

8 Next, set the SYSTOLIC ALARM SET HIGH knob. (The setting you choose will vary, depending on the doctor's orders.) If, at any time during the monitoring, your patient's systolic blood pressure reaches this setting, the monitor will sound an alarm.

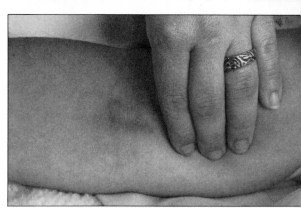

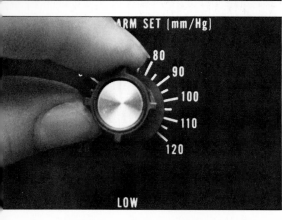

9 Now, set the SYSTOLIC ALARM SET LOW knob, as shown here. If the patient's systolic pressure falls to this level, predetermined by the doctor, the monitor sounds an alarm.

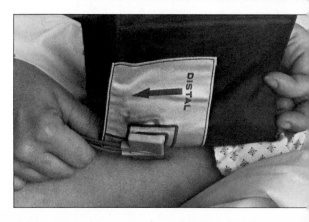

10 Attach the transducer to the pressure cuff. Use the outline traced on the pressure cuff to guide you. Since both the transducer's back and the appropriate section of the pressure cuff are covered with Velcro™, they'll adhere to each other securely.

11 Place a dime-sized daub of ultrasonic jelly on the front of each wing of the transducer, as shown here.

12 Now, locate the artery selected for monitoring. (For most adults, you'll choose the brachial artery. For an infant, you may choose a femoral or popliteal artery instead. But remember, an infant will require a different size cuff and transducer.)

In this photostory, we're using the patient's brachial artery. Locate it by palpating the patient's arm just above his antecubital space.

13 Now, place the transducer over the brachial artery, and firmly wrap the pressure cuff around the patient's arm. *Important:* Take care not to pinch a fold of skin under the pressure cuff.

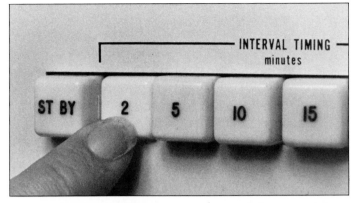

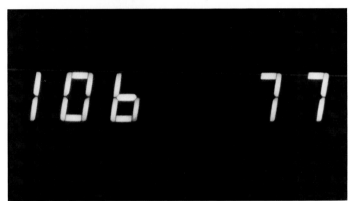

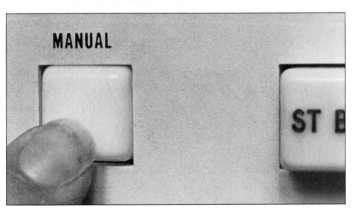

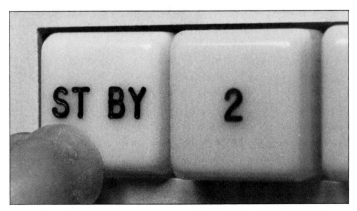

14 Look at the row of buttons labeled INTERVAL TIMING on the lower left side of the monitor's front. Push the appropriate button to tell the monitor how often to take a blood pressure reading. For example, suppose you want the monitor to take a reading every 2 minutes. Press the button marked *2*, as the nurse is doing here.

15 In this case, the monitor displays the patient's blood pressure every 2 minutes. Each blood pressure reading remains on the screen until the monitor records the next one.

16 If you decide to take a blood pressure reading between the predetermined intervals, simply push the MANUAL button, as shown here. The pressure cuff will inflate immediately, and the monitor will display the patient's blood pressure reading. Afterward, the monitor will continue to display the patient's blood pressure at the predetermined intervals.

17 To the left of the INTERVAL TIMING buttons, you'll see a button marked ST BY (stand by). If for some reason the blood pressure cuff doesn't deflate properly (or the patient complains that the pressure cuff's uncomfortably tight), push this button to deflate it. If the cuff didn't deflate properly, have the equipment serviced. But if the pressure was simply uncomfortable, reset the CUFF PRESSURE knob.

Arterial line

Dealing with complications of arterial lines

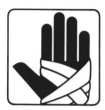

Whenever you manage an arterial line, stay alert for the first signs of complications. Read this chart to learn what to look for, how to respond, and how to reduce the risk of future complications.

Complication	Signs and symptoms	Possible causes
Thrombosis	• Loss or weakening of pulse below site • Loss of warmth, sensation, and mobility in limb below site • Damped or straight waveform on oscilloscope screen or readout strip	• Arterial damage during or after insertion • Sluggish flush solution flow rate • Failure to heparinize flush solution adequately • Failure to flush catheter routinely and after withdrawing blood samples • Irrigation of a clotted catheter with a syringe
Blood loss	• Bloody dressing; blood flowing from disconnected line.	• Dislodged catheter • Disconnected line
Air embolism	• Blood pressure drop • Rise in central venous pressure (CVP) • Weak, rapid pulse • Cyanosis • Loss of consciousness • Damped waveform	• Air in tubing • Loose connections
Systemic infection	• Sudden rise in patient's temperature and pulse rate • Chills and shaking • Blood pressure changes	• Poor aseptic technique • Contamination of equipment during manufacture, storage, or use • Irrigation of clogged catheter. (Irrigation may also cause an embolus.)
Arterial spasm	• Intermittent loss or weakening of pulse below insertion site • Irregular waveform on oscilloscope screen or readout strip	• Traumatic catheter insertion • Irritation of artery by catheter after insertion
Hematoma	• Swelling at insertion site, generalized swelling of limb • Bleeding at site	• Leakage of blood around catheter due to weakened or damaged artery • Failure to maintain pressure at site after catheter removal

Nursing intervention	Prevention tips
• Notify doctor. He may want to remove the line. Or he may perform an arteriotomy and Fogarty catheterization to remove the clot. • Document complication, as well as how you coped with it.	• Check patient's pulse immediately after catheter insertion, then once each hour. • Reduce trauma to artery by splinting limb and taping catheter securely. • Check flow rate hourly; maintain rate of 3 to 4 ml per hour. • Heparinize flush solution, according to hospital policy. • Flush catheter once every hour and after withdrawing blood samples. • Never irrigate an arterial catheter. You may flush a blood clot into the bloodstream.
• Stop the bleeding. • Check patient's vital signs. • Notify doctor if blood loss is great, and/or if patient's vital signs have changed. • If the line's disconnected, don't reconnect it. Instead, immediately replace contaminated equipment. • If the catheter's pulled out of the skin, apply direct pressure to the site, and notify doctor. • Check pulse and site frequently for signs of thrombosis or hematoma. • Document complication, as well as how you coped with it.	• Check line connections and insertion site frequently. • Tape catheter securely and splint limb.
• Turn the patient on his left side, and in Trendelenburg position. If air's entered his heart chambers, this position may keep the air on the right side of his heart. The pulmonary artery will then absorb small air bubbles. • Check the line for leaks. • Notify doctor immediately, and check vital signs. • Give patient oxygen, if ordered. • Document complication, as well as how you coped with it.	• Expel all air from the line before attaching it to the patient. • Make sure all connections are secure. Check connections routinely. • Change I.V. bag before it empties.
• Look for other sources of infection first. Get samples of urine, sputum, and blood for cultures, as ordered. • Notify doctor. He'll probably discontinue the line and send the equipment to the lab to be cultured.	• Review and improve aseptic technique. • Take care not to contaminate the site when bathing the patient. • If any part of the line's accidentally disconnected, don't rejoin it. Instead, replace the parts with sterile equipment.
• Notify doctor. • Prepare lidocaine hydrochloride. The doctor may inject it directly into the arterial catheter to relieve the spasm. *Important:* Make sure the lidocaine hydrochloride doesn't contain epinephrine, which could cause further arterial constriction. • Document complication, as well as how you coped with it.	• Tape the catheter securely to prevent it from moving in the artery. • Splint the patient's limb to stabilize the catheter.
• Stop the bleeding. • If the hematoma appears while the catheter's in place, notify doctor. • If the hematoma appears within ½ hour after catheter removal, apply ice to site. Otherwise, apply warm, moist compresses to help speed hematoma absorption. • Document complication, as well as how you coped with it.	• Tape catheter securely and splint limb to prevent damage to the artery. • After the catheter's removed, apply firm, manual pressure over site for about 10 minutes, until bleeding stops. Finally, apply a pressure bandage. (To learn how, see page 90.)

Arterial line

Recognizing common arterial waveforms

Below is a typical normal arterial blood pressure waveform. Note the rapid upstroke, clear dicrotic notch, and clear end diastole.

But when you monitor a critically ill patient's blood pressure, you'll probably see variations of this waveform. The information on this page will help you recognize and interpret other common arterial waveforms.

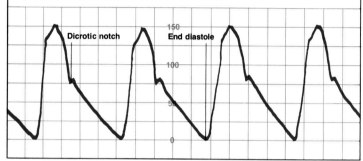

Dicrotic notch   **End diastole**

ALTERNATIONS OF HIGH AND LOW WAVES IN A REGULAR PATTERN

Possible cause
- Patient with ventricular bigeminy

Nursing action
- Check patient's EKG to confirm ventricular bigeminy. It should reflect premature ventricular contractions (PVCs) every second beat.

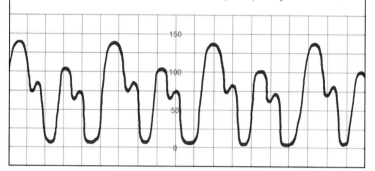

FLATTENED WAVEFORM

Possible cause
- Waveform damped, or patient hypotensive

Nursing action
- Check patient's blood pressure with a sphygmomanometer. If his pressure's very low or unobtainable, suspect hypotension.
- If you can obtain a blood pressure measurement with a sphygmomanometer, suspect damping. Troubleshoot the problem by flushing the line. (For other troubleshooting tips, see the chart on page 78.)

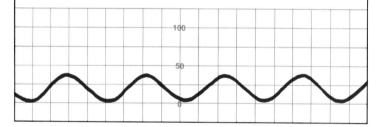

SLIGHTLY ROUNDED WAVEFORM, WITH CONSISTENT VARIATIONS IN SYSTOLIC HEIGHT

Possible cause
- Patient on ventilator, with positive end expiratory pressure (PEEP)

Nursing action
- Check patient's systolic blood pressure regularly. The difference between the highest and lowest systolic pressure should be less than 10 mm Hg. If the difference is greater than 10 mm Hg, suspect pulsus paradoxus, caused, for example, by cardiac tamponade.

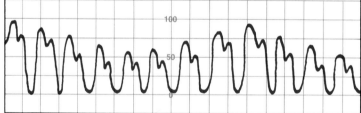

ERRATIC, RAGGED WAVEFORM

Possible cause
- Catheter tip movement in artery

Nursing action
- Stabilize the catheter by taping and splinting the insertion site.
- Notify doctor. He may try to reposition the catheter tip.

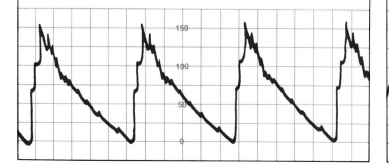

SLOW UPSTROKE

Possible cause
- Patient with aortic stenosis

Nursing action
- Check patient's heart sounds for signs of aortic stenosis. The doctor will document suspected aortic stenosis in his notes.

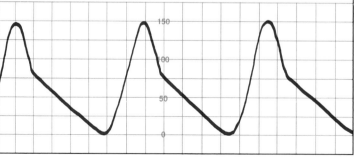

Pulmonary artery line

What's one of the most reliable methods for measuring your patient's cardiovascular and pulmonary functions? Most health-care professionals agree that right-sided heart catheterization can provide highly accurate information about his progress (or lack of it).

You may be familiar with the Swan-Ganz® balloon-tipped catheter made by American Edwards Laboratories. But because other companies make similar catheters, we'll call any catheter of this type a pulmonary artery (PA) catheter.

In the past, percutaneous PA catheter insertion was guided by fluoroscopy. But today, catheter insertion's guided by the same monitor that measures your patient's hemodynamic pressure. On the following pages, you'll see exactly how the waveform pinpoints catheter position.

After the PA catheter's in place, you can use it to monitor your patient's pulmonary artery pressure (PAP) and pulmonary artery wedge pressure (PAWP). As you'll discover in these pages, you can also use some PA catheters to measure cardiac output (CO) and central venous pressure (CVP). (Since you may also measure CVP with a fluid-filled manometer, we've included information on using a manometer, too.)

Consider your skills essential to your patient's health. Make sure they're sharp by studying what follows.

The pulmonary artery catheter: A close look

Pulmonary artery (PA) catheters are made of pliable, radiopaque polyvinylchloride. This catheter is about 43¼" (110 cm) long, marked in 10 cm increments. It has four lumens: a distal and a proximal lumen, which are fluid-filled for pressure monitoring; a thermistor lumen, which holds the wires connecting the thermistor to the cardiac output computer; and a balloon inflation lumen with valve. As a result, this catheter can measure several pressures, as well as cardiac output.

Important: Keep in mind that PA catheters vary, depending on the manufacturer. Consult the manufacturer's manual for details.

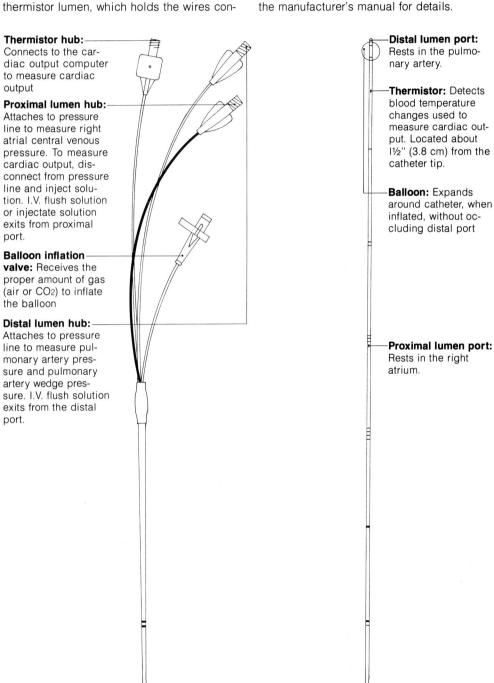

Thermistor hub: Connects to the cardiac output computer to measure cardiac output

Proximal lumen hub: Attaches to pressure line to measure right atrial central venous pressure. To measure cardiac output, disconnect from pressure line and inject solution. I.V. flush solution or injectate solution exits from proximal port.

Balloon inflation valve: Receives the proper amount of gas (air or CO_2) to inflate the balloon

Distal lumen hub: Attaches to pressure line to measure pulmonary artery pressure and pulmonary artery wedge pressure. I.V. flush solution exits from the distal port.

Distal lumen port: Rests in the pulmonary artery.

Thermistor: Detects blood temperature changes used to measure cardiac output. Located about 1½" (3.8 cm) from the catheter tip.

Balloon: Expands around catheter, when inflated, without occluding distal port

Proximal lumen port: Rests in the right atrium.

Pulmonary artery line

How to set up equipment for a pulmonary artery (PA) catheter

If the doctor's planning to insert a pulmonary artery (PA) catheter in your patient, he'll expect you to set up the monitoring equipment. Start by following the same procedure you used for a peripheral arterial line (see pages 82 to 87). Then, when the tubing, transducer dome, and stopcocks are completely flushed, set up the line in one of the ways shown below. Which setup you choose depends on the number of lines the doctor wants monitored.

As you set up the equipment, explain the procedure to your patient. Remember, he's probably apprehensive, so do your best to reassure him.

1 Let's imagine the doctor wants to monitor your patient's pulmonary artery pressure (PAP) and pulmonary artery wedge pressure (PAWP). To do so, he'll insert a PA catheter with only one lumen hub. In this illustration, you see a setup for this type of PA catheter.

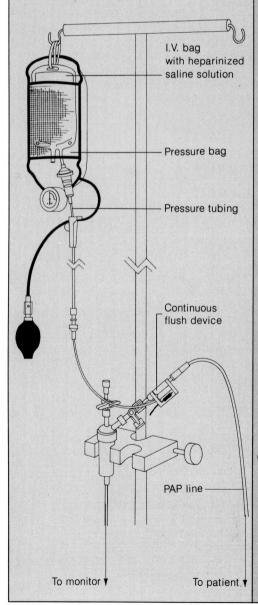

I.V. bag with heparinized saline solution

Pressure bag

Pressure tubing

Continuous flush device

PAP line

To monitor ▾   To patient ▾

2 But suppose the doctor also wants to monitor right atrial (RA) pressure (also called central venous pressure, or CVP). In that case, he'll insert a PA catheter with *two* lumen hubs. As you see in this illustration, you'll need a Y-connector between the I.V. bag and the transducer.

Mount a double stopcock manifold on the I.V. pole above the transducer, and connect each line's continuous flush device to a stopcock. To measure PAP or PAWP, turn the stopcock controlling the RA line off to the transducer and open the PAP line to the transducer, as shown here. To monitor RA pressure (CVP), reverse this procedure.

Important: As soon as you take an RA reading, close the RA line and reopen the PAP line. The doctor will expect you to monitor PAP continuously.

Can your monitor display two pressures at once? To get two pressure readings, you'll have to use two transducers. Connect the second transducer to the RA line.

If your patient has a peripheral arterial line in place (in addition to his PAP and RA lines), use a triple stopcock manifold. You'll use a three-way connector between the I.V. bag and the transducer, instead of a Y-connector.

Important: No matter which setup you use, you must level each transducer's balancing port with the patient's right atrium.

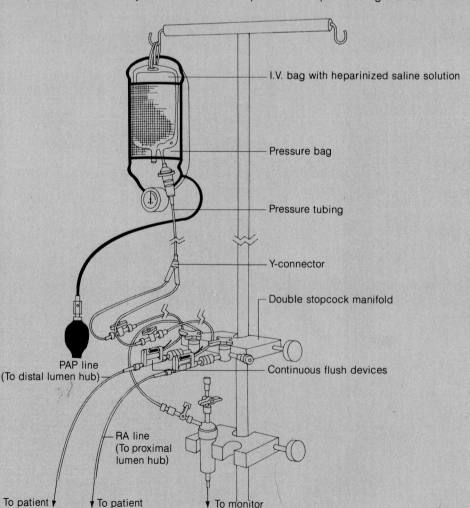

I.V. bag with heparinized saline solution

Pressure bag

Pressure tubing

Y-connector

Double stopcock manifold

Continuous flush devices

PAP line (To distal lumen hub)

RA line (To proximal lumen hub)

To patient ▾   ▾ To patient   ▾ To monitor

Pulmonary artery (PA) catheter insertion

After you've set up the monitoring equipment, the doctor may insert the pulmonary artery (PA) catheter percutaneously into your patient's median basilic vein. Or, he may choose the subclavian, internal jugular, or femoral vein instead, depending on the patient's condition. After insertion, he'll ease the catheter further into the patient's vein, until it passes through the right side of the heart and enters the pulmonary artery.

Examine these illustrations. They'll show you the route the catheter travels from the right atrium to the pulmonary artery. In addition, they'll show you how the monitor's waveform changes as the catheter progresses. The doctor depends on these waveforms to tell him the catheter tip's location. As he works, he'll expect you to record the pressure in each location.

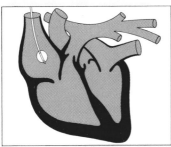

Right atrial (RA) pressure
Normal range
Mean: 3 to 6 mm Hg

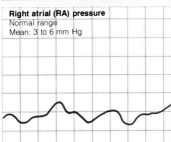

1 When the tip of the PA catheter reaches your patient's right atrium from the superior vena cava, the waveform on the oscilloscope screen or readout strip will look like this. When it does, the doctor will inflate the catheter's balloon, which will float the tip through the tricuspid valve and into the right ventricle.

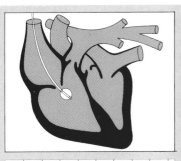

Right ventricular (RV) pressure
Normal range
Systolic: 17 to 32 mm Hg
Diastolic: 1 to 7 mm Hg

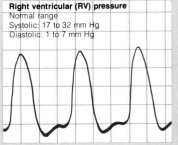

2 When the catheter tip reaches the patient's right ventricle, the waveform will look like this.

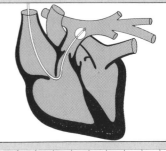

Pulmonary artery pressure (PAP)
Normal range
Systolic: 17 to 32 mm Hg
Diastolic: 4 to 13 mm Hg
Mean: 9 to 19 mm Hg

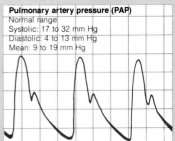

3 A waveform like this one indicates that the balloon has floated the catheter tip through the pulmonic valve into the pulmonary artery.

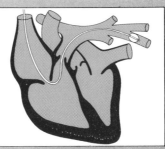

Pulmonary artery wedge pressure (PAWP)
Normal range
Mean: 8 to 12 mm Hg

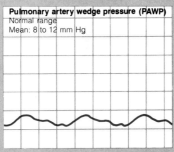

4 Blood flow in the pulmonary artery will then carry the catheter balloon into one of the pulmonary artery's many smaller branches. When the vessel becomes too narrow for the balloon to pass through, the balloon wedges in the vessel, occluding it. The monitor will then display a pulmonary artery wedge pressure (PAWP) waveform, like this one.

Note: This pressure is sometimes called pulmonary capillary wedge pressure (PCWP), or pulmonary artery occlusion pressure (PAOP).

At that point, the doctor will deflate the balloon. Without the inflated balloon to support it, the catheter tip will slip back into the main branch of the pulmonary artery, making the PAP waveform reappear (see the waveform in Step 3). Now, the catheter's placed correctly. The doctor will finish the procedure by securely suturing the catheter to the patient's skin.

Pulmonary artery line

Interpreting your patient's pulmonary artery pressure (PAP)

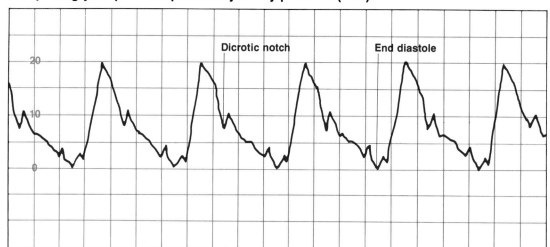

A typical pulmonary artery pressure (PAP) waveform looks like the one shown here. The normal PAP range is between 17 and 32 mm Hg systolic, 4 and 13 mm Hg diastolic, and 9 and 19 mm Hg mean.

Note the steep upstroke at the beginning of each wave. This upstroke indicates right ventricular ejection and the opening of the pulmonic valve. The dicrotic notch, visible on the downstroke, indicates closing of the pulmonic valve.

Your patient's PAP reflects venous pressure in his lungs, as well as mean filling pressure for the left side of his heart. In addition, a patient's PA systolic pressure usually equals his right ventricular (RV) systolic pressure (unless he suffers from pulmonary stenosis). Therefore, his PAP also reflects right ventricular function.

A rise in your patient's PAP may indicate one or more of the following:
- fluid overload
- left ventricular failure
- increased pulmonary blood flow
- pulmonary hypertension
- mitral stenosis.

Inflating a PA catheter's balloon

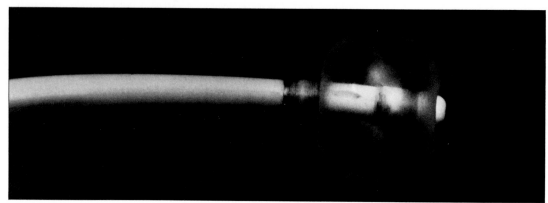

You'll inflate the balloon at the end of the pulmonary artery (PA) catheter when you take a pulmonary artery wedge pressure (PAWP) reading. In most cases, you'll inflate it with air. This is safe, even if the balloon ruptures, because the pulmonary artery will usually carry the escaping air bubbles to the lungs, where they're expelled.

But don't use air if escaping air bubbles could possibly enter your patient's arterial circulation (for example, if he has a suspected right to left intracardiac shunt). Instead, use CO_2. Why? Because CO_2 is 20 times more soluble than air in blood. A CO_2 bubble that escapes into an artery will probably dissolve before it can cause a dangerous embolism.

Never use liquid to inflate the catheter's balloon. If you do, the balloon won't float properly or deflate completely.

Important: Make sure the balloon's completely deflated at all times, except when you take a PAWP reading. Otherwise, the balloon may wedge in a branch of the pulmonary artery. And prolonged wedging, as you know, may cause a pulmonary infarction.

PAWP: What it tells you

When the pulmonary artery (PA) catheter tip is positioned properly in your patient's artery, you can inflate its flexible latex balloon to measure his pulmonary artery wedge pressure (PAWP). This helps you determine his left ventricular function.

On the opposite page, we'll show you how to take a PAWP measurement. Here's what happens during the procedure.

After the inflated balloon occludes a pulmonary artery branch, the catheter's distal lumen, located in front of the balloon, registers left heart pressure. This PAWP measurement will give you an accurate picture of your patient's left heart function.

Record the mean PAWP displayed on the monitor and immediately deflate the balloon. When the balloon's deflated, the catheter tip will float back into the main branch of the pulmonary artery.

In most cases, the doctor will not order PAWP readings to be taken more than once every 4 hours. More frequent inflations could rupture the balloon.

Measuring your patient's pulmonary artery wedge pressure (PAWP)

1 *In this photo-story, we'll show you how to measure your patient's pulmonary artery wedge pressure (PAWP). The only equipment you'll need is a tuberculin (TB) syringe. Follow these steps:*

Wash your hands thoroughly before you begin. Then, place your patient on her back or in semi-Fowler's position, explaining the procedure to her as you do.

If necessary, balance and calibrate the equipment. Remember to position the transducer's balancing port level with the patient's right atrium.

[Inset] Press the mean pressure button (M) on the monitor.

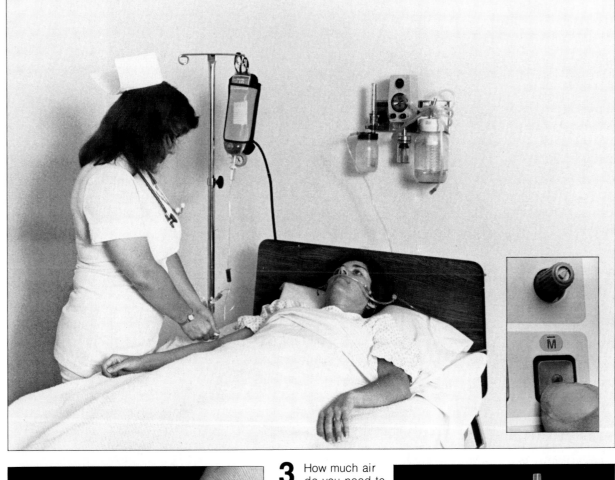

2 Pull the pigtail on the continuous flush device to flush the line. If the line doesn't flush properly, locate the problem, and correct it before you continue. (For troubleshooting tips, see page 79.)

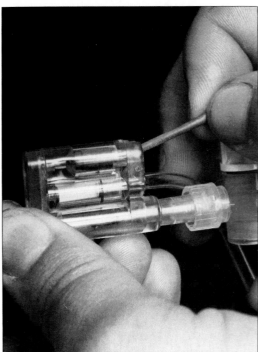

3 How much air do you need to inflate the balloon? Chances are, less than 1 cc. Check the side of the catheter for the *maximum* amount recommended by the manufacturer. Then, draw 0.3 to 0.5 cc less than that amount into the syringe.

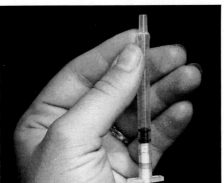

4 Make sure the balloon inflation valve on the PA catheter is open, and attach the syringe to it.

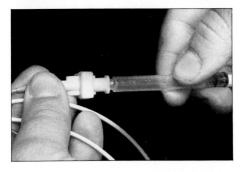

Pulmonary artery line

Measuring your patient's pulmonary artery wedge pressure (PAWP) continued

5 To inflate the balloon with air, slowly and carefully depress the syringe plunger. (You'll feel slight resistance as you do.) *Important:* If you don't feel resistance, suspect a ruptured balloon, and stop the procedure immediately.

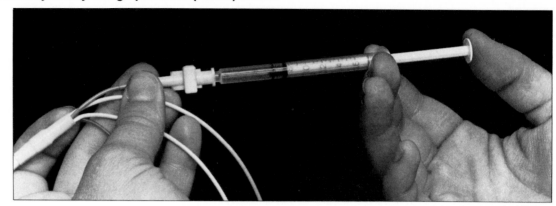

6 As you inflate the balloon, watch the oscilloscope screen closely. Stop injecting air as soon as the pulmonary artery pressure (PAP) waveform changes to a PAWP waveform, as shown here. This indicates that the balloon's wedged in a narrow branch of the pulmonary artery.

Record the digital PAWP reading displayed on the monitor.

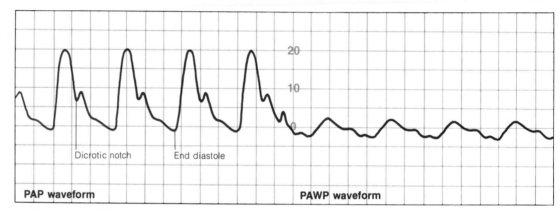

Dicrotic notch   End diastole

PAP waveform   PAWP waveform

7 Then, immediately remove the syringe, as shown here, and let the air escape from the inflation valve by itself. *Important:* Never aspirate the air with the syringe. You may rupture the balloon.

When the balloon deflates completely, the PAP waveform will return.

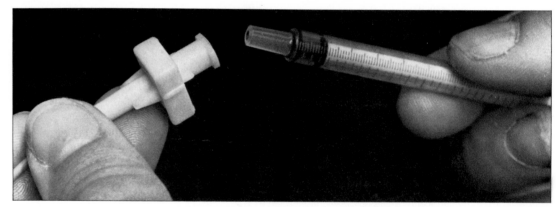

8 What if a PAWP waveform, like the one shown here, remains on the oscilloscope screen? The balloon may still be inflated, or the catheter tip may have become wedged in a small pulmonary capillary. Ask the patient to cough, which may jolt the catheter tip free. But if a clear PAP waveform doesn't return, notify the doctor at once, and prepare the patient for a chest X-ray. *Remember:* Prolonged wedging may cause a pulmonary infarction.

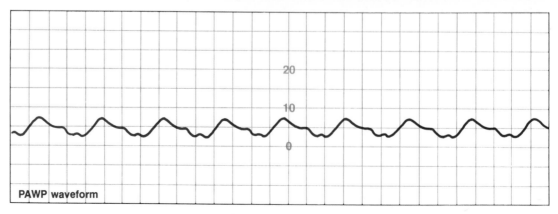

PAWP waveform

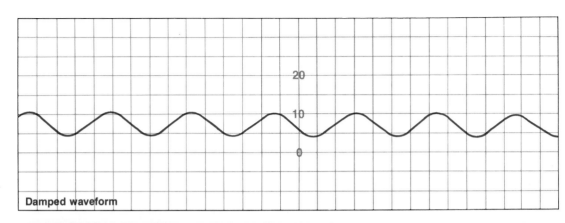

Damped waveform

9 Suppose a damped PAP waveform appears on the oscilloscope screen. In this case, the balloon may still be partially inflated. Try to restore a clear PAP waveform by flushing the line. If that doesn't work, notify the doctor.

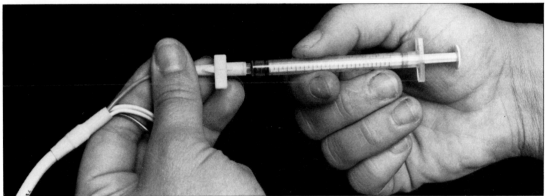

10 When you're sure the balloon's completely deflated, depress the syringe plunger to expel all air from the syringe, and once again attach the syringe to the balloon inflation valve. This precaution ensures that no one will mistake the balloon inflation valve for an injection hub.

Document the entire procedure, including the PAWP reading, in your nurses' notes and patient's chart.

Interpreting your patient's pulmonary artery wedge pressure (PAWP)

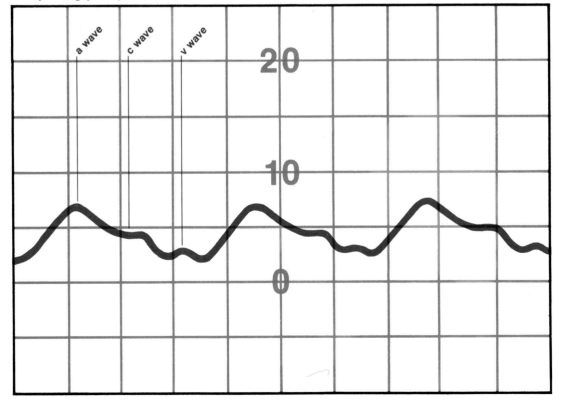

This illustration shows a normal PAWP waveform. The normal PAWP range is between 8 and 12 mm Hg, and approximates pulmonary artery (PA) diastolic pressure. Notify the doctor if the difference between PAWP and PA diastolic pressure is greater than 5 mm Hg.

A rise in your patient's PAWP may indicate one or more of the following:
* left ventricular failure
* fluid overload
* pulmonary hypertension
* mitral stenosis
* mitral insufficiency.

a wave. Left atrium contracts. Corresponds to EKG's P wave.
c wave. Tricuspid valve closes. (Because wave pressure is so low at this point, you may not be able to see the c wave.)
v wave. Left ventricle contracts; mitral valve bulges into left atrium. Corresponds to EKG's T wave.

Pulmonary artery line

Thermodilution technique: How it works

As you know, the term cardiac output indicates the amount of blood ejected from the heart each minute. At rest, a healthy heart ejects from 4 to 6 liters each minute.

If your patient's pulmonary artery (PA) catheter has a thermistor, you can measure his cardiac output with a special computer, using the thermodilution technique shown in the following photostory. These measurements will help you assess left ventricular and valve functions.

How does the thermodilution technique work? First, you'll inject a solution of known temperature and known volume into the patient's cardiovascular system through the proximal lumen of the PA catheter. This solution will then mix with the blood of the superior vena cava or right atrium (depending on the PA catheter's exact location) and lower the temperature of the blood in the heart. When this cooler blood flows past the thermistor embedded in the distal end of the PA catheter, the thermistor will detect the temperature drop and send a signal back to the computer. Finally, the computer will analyze this information and record the patient's cardiac output on its display screen.

What kind of solution do you inject, and at what temperature? Use either normal saline solution or 5% dextrose in water. Make sure it's cooler than the patient's blood temperature. In most cases, a room temperature solution cools the blood adequately for an accurate measurement. But if your equipment doesn't register precisely, or your patient has wide respiratory fluctuations, use solution iced to 32° to 39.2° F. (0° to 4° C.) instead. Why? Because iced solution will reduce the temperature of blood in the heart even more, causing the thermistor to send a stronger signal to the computer. As a result, your cardiac output measurement may be more accurate.

Measuring cardiac output with the thermodilution technique

1 *Planning to set up equipment for the thermodilution technique? Before you begin, check the monitor's waveform to make sure the pulmonary artery (PA) catheter is positioned properly in the pulmonary artery and the balloon's completely deflated. If you're uncertain about either, notify the doctor and prepare the patient for an X-ray. But if everything's OK, follow these steps:*

Obtain a cardiac output computer (the one shown here is made by American Edwards Laboratories). Make sure it contains a fully charged battery. In addition, gather the equipment shown in the photo below: 500 ml bag 5% dextrose in water (warmed to room temperature), five 10 cc syringes with needles, a container for the injectate bath, and a computer probe with cable. *Note:* If you're planning to use iced injectate solution, get ice as well.

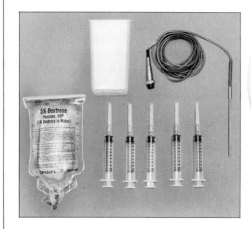

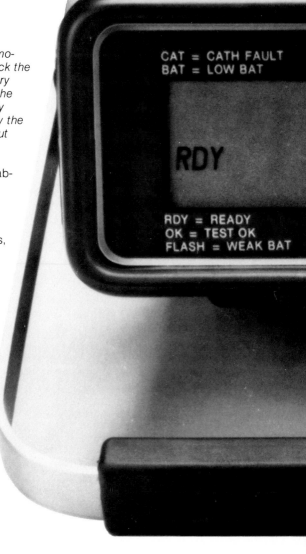

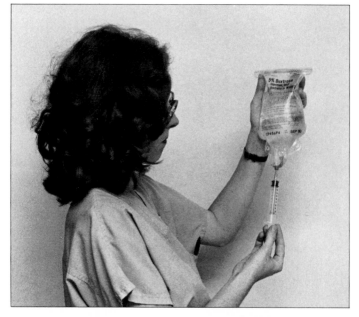

2 Using aseptic technique, fill one of the syringes with 10 ml of 5% dextrose in water, as the nurse is doing here.

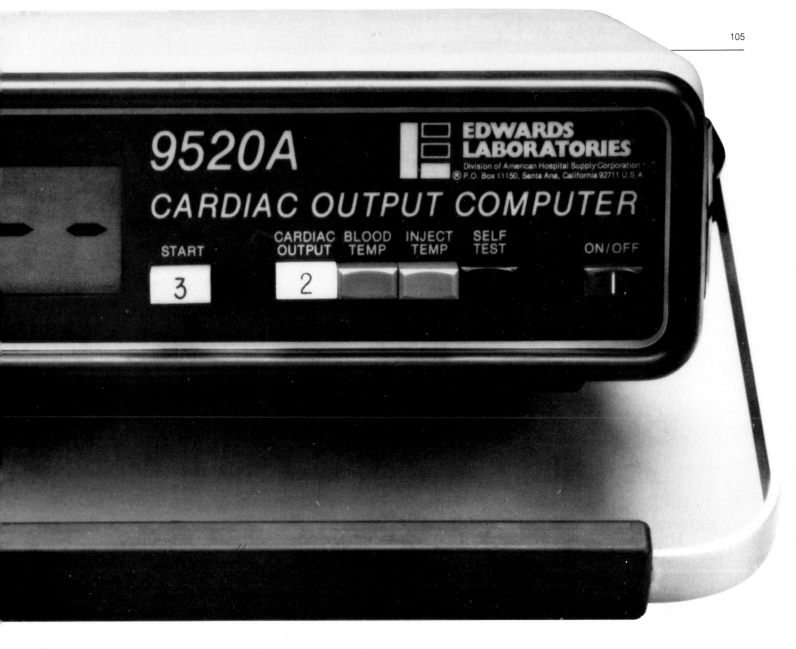

9520A
EDWARDS LABORATORIES
Division of American Hospital Supply Corporation
® P.O. Box 11150, Santa Ana, California 92711 U.S.A.

CARDIAC OUTPUT COMPUTER

START — CARDIAC OUTPUT — BLOOD TEMP — INJECT TEMP — SELF TEST — ON/OFF

3   2

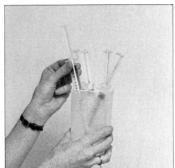

3 Cap the needle, and place it in the injectate bath container, with the barrel up. Repeat steps 2 and 3 until all five syringes are filled, capped, and resting in the container.

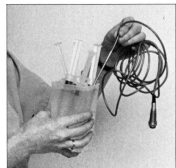

4 With your scissors, cut open the 500 ml bag 5% dextrose in water and fill the container. Now, the syringes filled with injectate solution (5% dextrose in water) are bathed in a room temperature bath of the same solution. Put the computer probe into the injectate bath, as shown here.

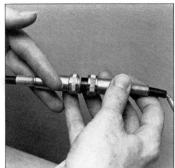

5 Next, look at the cable attached to the back of the computer. Notice that it's divided into two branches, one marked INJECTATE PROBE and the other marked CATHETER. Connect the computer probe's cable to the branch marked INJECTATE PROBE. Screw them together tightly.

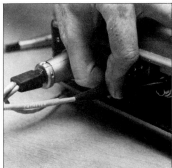

6 Then, take the branch marked CATHETER and plug it into the receptacle to the right of the computer cable receptacle.

Pulmonary artery line

Measuring cardiac output with the thermodilution technique continued

7 Depress the ON/OFF button on the front of the computer. Wait several seconds. When you see *RDY* (ready) on the computer screen, you're ready to begin the self-test pro-

cedure. This procedure will help you tell if the cable and computer are functioning properly. Push the SELF TEST button, and look for a series of dashes on the computer screen.

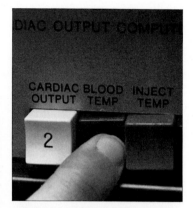

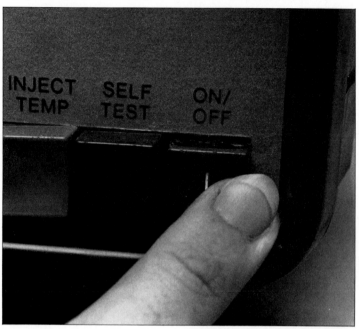

10 Push the BLOOD TEMP button on the front of the computer, and watch for the patient's blood temperature to be displayed on the screen. Compare this blood temperature with his predetermined body temperature. If they differ by more than *0.3°*, suspect a faulty thermistor in the catheter tip, and notify the doctor.

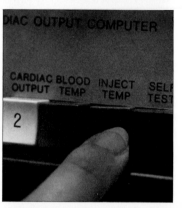

11 Next, push the INJECT TEMP button, and watch for the temperature of the injectate bath to be displayed on the screen. When the computer later measures your patient's cardiac output, it will use both the patient's blood temperature and the injectate bath temperature in its calculations.

8 Then, push the START button. First, you'll see *0.00* on the screen. If all's well, you'll see *OK* several seconds later. (If you see another series of dashes instead, get another computer.)

Wait about 30 seconds until you see *RDY* on the screen.
☙ *Nursing tip:* For additional assurance that the equipment's functioning properly, press the BLOOD TEMP button. The computer should display a 37° C. reading (plus or minus 1°).

9 Remove the cable branch marked CATHETER from its receptacle, and connect it to the thermistor hub of the patient's pulmonary artery (PA) catheter. *Note:* If *CAT* appears on the screen after you make this connection, tighten all connections from the computer to the patient. If *CAT* still shows on the screen, suspect a faulty circuit in the catheter. Consult the manufacturer's manual for further instructions.

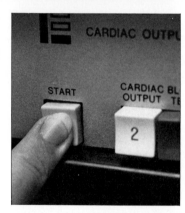

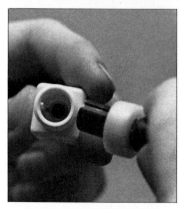

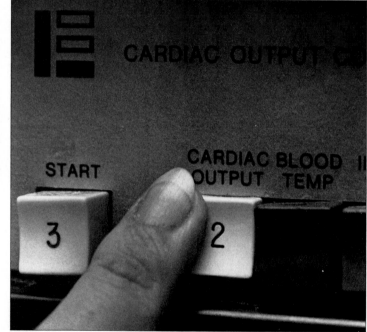

12 Now, the computer's ready to measure your patient's cardiac output. Push the CARDIAC OUTPUT button on the computer, and wait for

RDY to appear on the screen.
Then, push the START button. Quickly, take one of the syringes from the injectate bath and remove the capped needle.

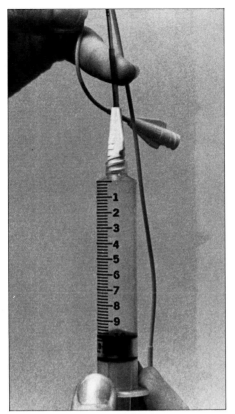

13 Attach the syringe to the catheter's proximal lumen hub. Then, immediately inject the injectate solution into the catheter at a rate of at least 10 ml every 4 seconds. *Remember:* The injectate solution will begin to change temperature as soon as you remove it from the injectate bath. To ensure an accurate reading, avoid spreading your fingers over the syringe, because this will warm the solution.

In about 15 seconds, expect the computer to display the patient's cardiac output in liters per minute. The computer will continue to display this figure until you inject more solution.

When *RDY* appears on the computer screen, remove another syringe from the injectate bath. Inject more solution (using the same procedure).

Nursing tip: Do you suspect the computer's cardiac output readings are inaccurate? Try replacing the battery. A low battery may pass the self-test procedure, yet still produce false readings.

Repeat the procedure, as the doctor orders. Most likely, he'll want you to take at least three cardiac output measurements and average them. The average measurement is the patient's cardiac output for that particular time.

Understanding central venous pressure (CVP)

How does measuring right atrial central venous pressure (CVP) help you assess your patient's condition? CVP tells you the pressure and volume of blood returning to the right atrium through the subclavian vein. Since it accurately measures right atrial blood pressure, which in turn reflects right ventricular blood pressure, CVP tells you how well the right side of the heart functions.

However, CVP is a poor indicator of how well the *left* side of your patient's heart functions. For this reason, the doctor may prefer to insert a multiple-lumen pulmonary artery (PA) catheter, rather than a single-lumen catheter placed in the superior vena cava. A PA catheter can measure both right- and left-side heart functions.

How do you measure CVP?

No matter which type of catheter your patient has in place, you can monitor his CVP in two ways: either with a transducer and monitor, or with a fluid-filled manometer. If your patient has a PA catheter in place, connect the PA catheter's *proximal lumen hub* to the transducer or to the manometer. (Remember, the PA catheter's proximal lumen port lies in the patient's right atrium, the best location for measuring CVP.)

Unlike the transducer and monitor, which measure CVP in millimeters of mercury (mm Hg), a manometer measures CVP in centimeters of water (cm H_2O). If the doctor changes your patient's monitoring setup from a transducer and monitor to a manometer (or vice versa), you'll need to know how to convert the measurements. Otherwise, you'll be unable to tell if your patient's CVP changes significantly. Keep these formulas in a handy place:
- To convert cm H_2O to mm Hg: cm $H_2O \div 1.36 =$ mm Hg
- To convert mm Hg to cm H_2O: mm Hg x 1.36 = cm H_2O

For details on measuring CVP with a manometer, see the photostory on the following page.

CVP lines: Some special considerations

Let's imagine the doctor inserts a single-lumen central venous pressure (CVP) line percutaneously into one of your patient's large central veins; for example, the subclavian or internal jugular. Because the vein is so large, take special precautions before, during, and after insertion. Here are some guidelines:

• Assemble sterile equipment, including a radiopaque catheter. Remember to maintain sterile technique throughout the entire insertion procedure.

• Position your patient in a 30° Trendelenburg position, with a rolled towel placed lengthwise between his shoulders. This will encourage the large central vein to distend, making catheter insertion easier.

• Ask the patient to bear down (Valsalva maneuver) as the doctor punctures the vein. By increasing intrathoracic pressure, the Valsalva maneuver counteracts strong negative pressure from the vein. As a result, an air embolus is less likely.

• After insertion, make sure the doctor orders an X-ray to confirm proper catheter placement in the superior vena cava or right atrium.

• Make sure all connections in the line are secure. As you know, a loose connection may cause an air embolus.

• When you take readings, place the patient flat on his back, without a pillow, if possible. But adjust the position if he's uncomfortable. Then, make sure he's in the same position for all readings. Document it so the next nurse who takes a reading will place him the same way. By taking all readings under the same conditions, you'll be able to recognize significant changes. *Note:* Never position the patient so his legs dangle over the edge of the bed. Doing so will produce a false low reading.

• Establish a baseline CVP range by taking initial readings 15, 30, and 60 minutes apart. Then, if a CVP reading varies by more than 2 cm H_2O (1 mm Hg) from the baseline, notify the doctor.

• Replace each container of I.V. solution before it runs dry. Otherwise, negative pressure from the vein may pull air from the container into the patient, causing an air embolus.

• Keep the insertion site clean and dry to minimize the risk of infection. Replace the patient's dressing every 48 hours, or whenever it becomes wet or soiled.

• Routinely replace the entire setup every 48 hours to minimize the risk of infection. Also, immediately replace any disconnected equipment. Never reconnect it.

Pulmonary artery line

Measuring CVP with a manometer

1 *In this photostory, you'll see how to take a central venous pressure (CVP) reading with a manometer. To do this properly, you'll need a manometer, an I.V. pole, a container of I.V. solution (as ordered by the doctor), manometer tubing, and I.V. tubing. Because a single-lumen catheter placed in the superior vena cava won't encounter strong pressures from the left side of the heart, you won't need rigid pressure tubing, a continuous flush device, or a pressure bag. Set up the equipment while the doctor performs the insertion.*

The manometer we're featuring has two parts: a reusable metal scale and disposable tubing with a three-way stopcock attached. Clamp the metal scale to the I.V. pole so the scale is vertical, as shown here. Then, spike and hang the I.V. container and prime the tubing. Hang the I.V. container 30" to 36" (76.2 to 90 cm) above the insertion site. If you hang it lower, the infusion won't flow properly, allowing blood to back up in the catheter.

2 After attaching the stopcock on the manometer's tubing to the bottom of the scale, stretch the tubing to the top of the manometer column and insert it in the brackets, as shown here. Then, connect the I.V. tubing to the open side of the stopcock.

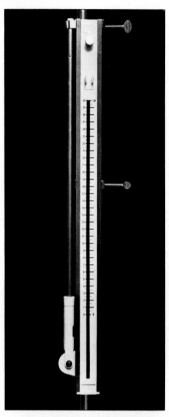

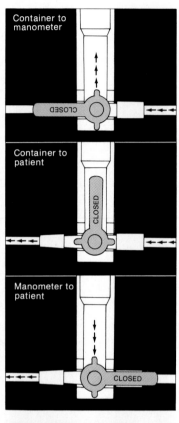

Container to manometer

Container to patient

Manometer to patient

3 Examine the three stopcock positions shown here. You'll use these positions to control fluid flow through the CVP line.

4 Turn the stopcock to CONTAINER-TO-MANOMETER position, as shown here. Fill the manometer column with I.V. solution until it's almost full. (Don't fill it to the top, or you'll contaminate the manometer's air filter.)

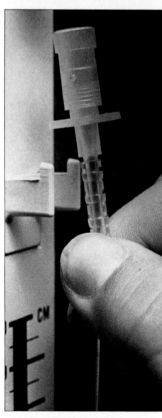

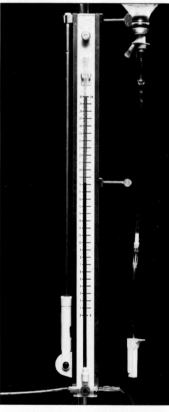

5 Now, turn the stopcock to CONTAINER-TO-PATIENT position, and flush the tubing. When all the air's expelled, close the I.V. tubing's flow clamp. Now, the doctor will connect the patient's catheter to this tubing.

Open the flow clamp and adjust the I.V. flow rate, as ordered by the doctor.

6 Position the patient flat on his back. Lower the manometer's leveling arm, as shown here, and line up the *zero mark* on the manometer scale with the patient's right atrium. (Mark this spot with adhesive tape, and take all subsequent CVP readings from this level.)

To take a CVP reading, turn the stopcock to MANOMETER-TO-PATIENT position. The fluid will drop in the manometer column, stopping when the pressure equals that of the patient's CVP.

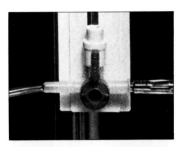

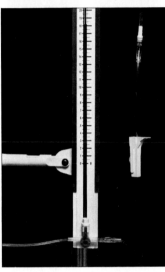

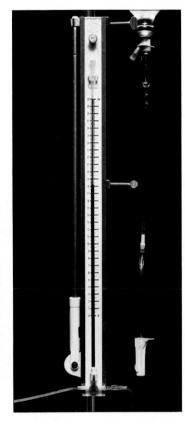

7 To eliminate bubbles, lightly tap the manometer column. Then, stand at eye level with the top of the fluid column. Expect the fluid column to rise and fall slightly as the patient breathes. Note the highest level the fluid reaches, and take your reading from the base of the meniscus.

Maintain catheter patency by returning the stopcock to CONTAINER-TO-PATIENT position as soon as you take your reading. Finally, adjust the flow rate and document the procedure. (For more details on how to take CVP measurements with a manometer, read the Nursing80 PHOTOBOOK *Managing I.V. Therapy.*)

Interpreting a right atrial CVP waveform

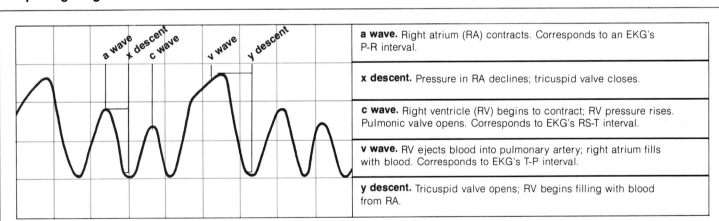

a wave. Right atrium (RA) contracts. Corresponds to an EKG's P-R interval.
x descent. Pressure in RA declines; tricuspid valve closes.
c wave. Right ventricle (RV) begins to contract; RV pressure rises. Pulmonic valve opens. Corresponds to EKG's RS-T interval.
v wave. RV ejects blood into pulmonary artery; right atrium fills with blood. Corresponds to EKG's T-P interval.
y descent. Tricuspid valve opens; RV begins filling with blood from RA.

If your patient has a pulmonary artery (PA) catheter in place, you'll probably monitor his right atrial CVP by connecting the catheter's proximal lumen hub to a transducer and monitor. Since the PA catheter's proximal port lies in the right atrium (RA), the monitor will display an RA waveform like the one shown here.

The normal range for RA pressure (the mean pressure in the right atrium during diastole) is from 3 to 6 mm Hg (5 to 15 cm H₂O).

RA pressure reflects right ventricular end diastolic pressure (RVEDP).

A drop in RA pressure, on the one hand, may indicate hypovolemia, vasodilation, or peripheral blood pooling.

A rise in RA pressure, on the other hand, may indicate one or more of the following:
• right ventricular (RV) failure

• left ventricular (LV) failure
• hypervolemia
• tricuspid valve stenosis or regurgitation
• constrictive pericarditis
• pulmonary hypertension
• air embolism
• vasoconstriction
• early cardiac tamponade.

Left atrial line

How does the doctor assess your patient's left atrial pressure (LAP)? In most cases, he'll probably measure it indirectly by taking a pulmonary artery wedge pressure (PAWP), as shown on page 104. But if your patient undergoes open heart surgery, the doctor may insert a small plastic catheter directly into his left atrium during surgery. After it's connected to a monitor and transducer postoperatively, the catheter will then enable the doctor to directly and accurately assess the patient's left atrial pressure during recovery.

What does LAP tell the doctor? Unless your patient has mitral valve disease, LAP is a reliable indicator of left ventricular end diastolic pressure (LVEDP), and therefore, left ventricular function. LAP is recorded at the end of atrial diastole, just before the mitral valve opens and empties blood into the ventricles.

Your responsibilities during the monitoring of LAP include setting up the equipment so it's ready for the patient as soon as he returns from surgery. On the next few pages, you'll see how.

Setting up a left atrial monitoring line

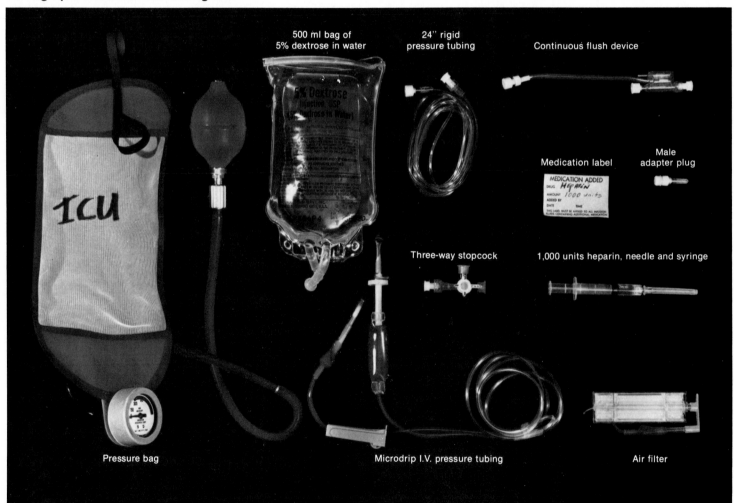

500 ml bag of 5% dextrose in water

24" rigid pressure tubing

Continuous flush device

Medication label

Male adapter plug

MEDICATION ADDED
DRUG *HEPARIN*
AMOUNT *1000 units*
ADDED BY
DATE   TIME

Three-way stopcock

1,000 units heparin, needle and syringe

Pressure bag

Microdrip I.V. pressure tubing

Air filter

1 *If the doctor inserted a catheter directly into your patient's left atrium during open heart surgery, he'll expect you to set up the monitoring equipment. Begin by washing your hands thoroughly. Remember to maintain strict aseptic technique throughout the procedure. Then, follow these steps:*

Gather the equipment shown in this photo, as well as a hemodynamic monitor, an I.V. pole, a transducer, and a transducer dome. For safety, use 5% dextrose in water as a flush solution, instead of normal saline solution. Why? Because an accidental overload of saline solution is more dangerous to an already compromised heart than an overload of 5% dextrose in water.

For your patient's additional safety, attach an air filter to the line. Remember, an air bubble pumped into your patient's left atrium may be fatal.

Turn on the monitor and plug in the transducer, so they can warm up. (If you plan to attach the line to a stopcock manifold, like one of those shown on page 98, make sure all the stopcocks and tubing are flushed ahead of time.)

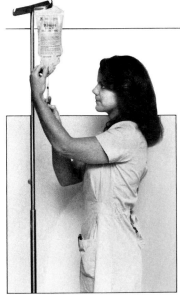

2 Hang the bag of 5% dextrose in water on the I.V. pole. Inject the heparin into the bag.

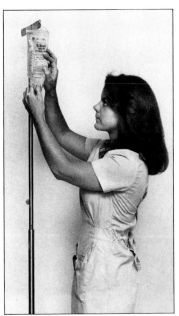

3 Place the properly filled out medication label on the bag, as the nurse is doing here.

Then, spike the bag and take it off the I.V. pole. Open the flow clamp, and squeeze out all air in the bag through the drip chamber.

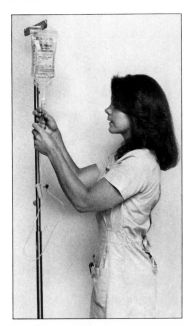

4 Hang the bag again, and close the flow clamp. Tilting the drip chamber slightly, *gently* squeeze it until it's half filled with solution, as the nurse is doing here. *Important:* Don't squeeze too forcibly or you may cause turbulence in the solution, producing air bubbles.

Next, open the flow clamp and prime the tubing. When all the air's expelled from the tubing, close the clamp.

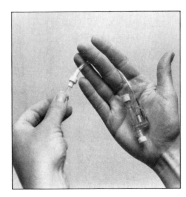

5 Attach the continuous flush device to the line, and flush it completely to expel air bubbles.

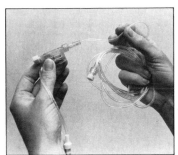

6 Next, attach the 24" pressure tubing to the continuous flush device. (This will give the patient some freedom of movement and prevent strain on the catheter.) Flush the pressure tubing.

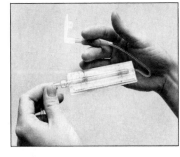

7 Now, attach the air filter to the end of the pressure tubing, as shown here. Flush the air filter by pulling the pigtail on the continuous flush device. Let the filter fill completely with fluid. *Important:* Make sure the filter's completely saturated with solution by letting it rest for several minutes; then, flush it again.

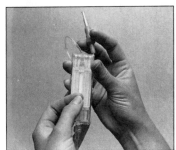

8 Now, rotate the filter from front to back, and check for air bubbles. If you see any, gently tap the filter as you continue to flush it, as the nurse is doing here. *Important:* Make sure all air's expelled from every part of the line. Otherwise, the pressure bag may force an air bubble into the patient's left atrium, causing an embolism.

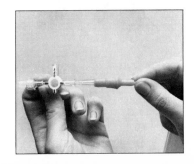

9 When all the air's expelled, continue flushing the tubing and attach the three-way stopcock. Then, completely flush the stopcock. *Note:* The clear protective cap you see on the end of the stopcock's lateral port guards against touch contamination. However, it's not airtight, so you can flush fluid through it.

Left atrial line

Setting up a left atrial monitoring line continued

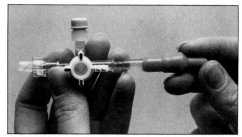

10 When the stopcock's flushed, cap the middle port with a male adapter plug (nipple port), and turn off the line to the air filter, as shown here.

11 Place the bag of 5% dextrose in water inside the pressure bag and inflate the pressure bag to 300 mm Hg, as the nurse is doing in the photo on the right. Now, you're ready to connect the line to the patient's catheter.
   Open the stopcock on the patient's cathe-ter so fluid drips slowly from the stopcock's lateral port. (If the patient's catheter was connected to another infusion line in the OR, his catheter will probably drip I.V. fluid. If not, it will probably drip blood.)
   Now, open the air filter stopcock's lateral port, so it drips I.V. solution, and connect it to the stopcock on the patient's catheter. Connecting the line when both ports are dripping fluid reduces the risk of trapping an air bubble.

12 If you're not attaching the line to a stopcock manifold, attach the trans-ducer dome to the continuous flush device, flush the dome, and attach the dome to the transducer. Then, mount the transducer on the I.V. pole, as shown here.

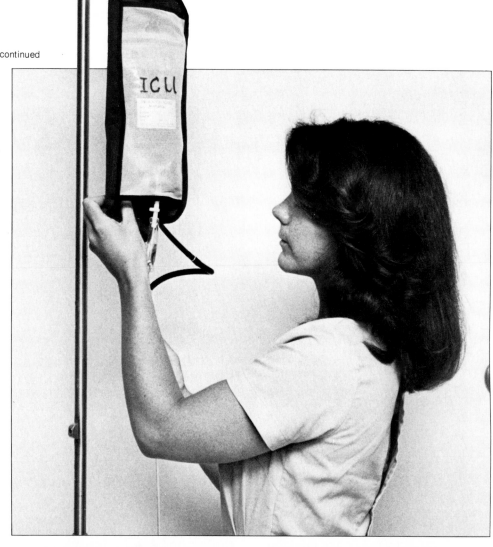

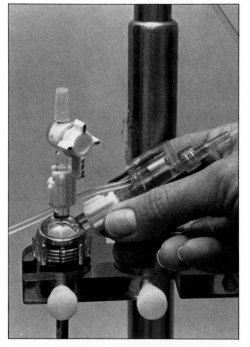

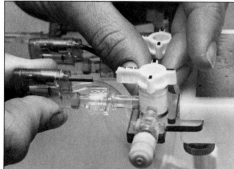

13 But most likely, you'll attach the line to a stopcock manifold, like the one you see here. No matter which system you use, remember that the transducer's balancing port must be level with the pa-tient's right atrium.
   Document the procedure thoroughly in your nurses' notes. Label the I.V. bag with your patient's name and room number; type and amount of I.V. solution; heparin dose; drip rate of the I.V. solution; the date and time you hung the bag; and your name.

How to evaluate LAP readings

The normal range for left atrial pressure (LAP) readings is 8 to 12 mm Hg, although readings vary from patient to patient. To establish a baseline reading for *your* patient, take an initial series of readings 15, 30, and 60 minutes after you begin monitoring him. Then, notify the doctor if any subsequent readings rise or fall more than 2 mm Hg.

Always take readings on the monitor's *mean* mode. By themselves, systolic and diastolic readings aren't significant.

In addition, take LAP readings at the end of exhalation. Normally, your patient's LAP will drop during inspiration (because of the drop in intrathoracic pressure), then rise back to baseline during exhalation. But if your patient's mechanically ventilated, expect his LAP to *rise* during inspiration, then *drop* back to baseline during exhalation.

Note: Is your patient on positive end expiratory pressure (PEEP)? Because PEEP continues to apply positive pressure to the patient's airways at the end of exhalation, expect his LAP to show a false high.

How to interpret an LAP waveform

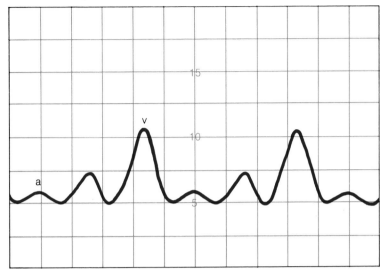

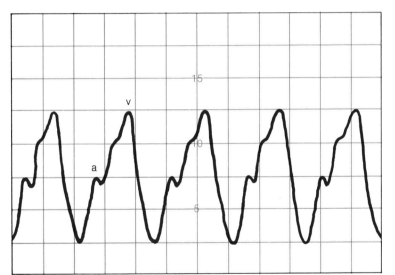

1 *What do left atrial pressure (LAP) waveforms look like?* These two illustrations show two LAP waveforms you're likely to see.

The illustration to the left shows a typical LAP waveform. At the point marked *a* on this waveform, the patient's left atrium contracts and his mitral valve closes. At the point marked *v,* his left ventricle contracts, his mitral valve opens, and his left ventricle begins filling.

2 You'll probably see an LAP waveform like this if your patient has mitral valve insufficiency. The heightened *v* waves indicate regurgitative blood during ventricular contraction.

Heightened *v* waves, accompanied by a rise of 2 mm Hg or more in LAP, may also indicate that the catheter's slipped through the mitral valve. Notify the doctor at once, so he can reposition the catheter.

Suppose this situation occurs in a patient who's had a mitral valve replacement. Auscultate his heart sounds. If the catheter's slipped through the prosthetic mitral valve, you won't be able to hear the valve click.

Care guidelines for the patient on LAP monitoring

To give your patient the full benefit of left atrial pressure (LAP) monitoring, while minimizing the risks, perform these procedures routinely:

• Balance and calibrate the monitoring equipment at least once every 8 hours.

• Observe the LAP waveform carefully, and take readings hourly. Thoroughly document all observations and readings in your nurses' notes and on the flow chart.

🕭 *Nursing tip:* To ensure accurate interpretation of values, take LAP readings at the same time you measure your patient's blood pressure, heart rate, right atrial central venous pressure, pulmonary artery pressure (PAP), and urinary output.

• Auscultate your patient's heart sounds at least once every 4 hours, or whenever you see a significant (2 mm Hg) change in LAP or waveform. Notify the doctor of any significant change.

• Change the dressing at the insertion site daily. Remove the dressing, and clean the site with povodine-iodine skin prep, observing strict aseptic technique. Check for redness, drainage, or broken sutures. If you see any of these problems, notify the doctor.

If all's well, redress the site with a precut tracheostomy dressing so the catheter doesn't kink. Then, tape the dressing securely in place.

• Replace the tubing as far as the filter once every 48 hours or more often, depending on your hospital's policy.

• Stay alert for common monitoring problems, and try to solve them. For troubleshooting tips, see pages 78 and 79. *Important:* If the catheter clots, *do not* attempt to fast flush it or to aspirate the clot with a syringe. Instead, notify the doctor at once.

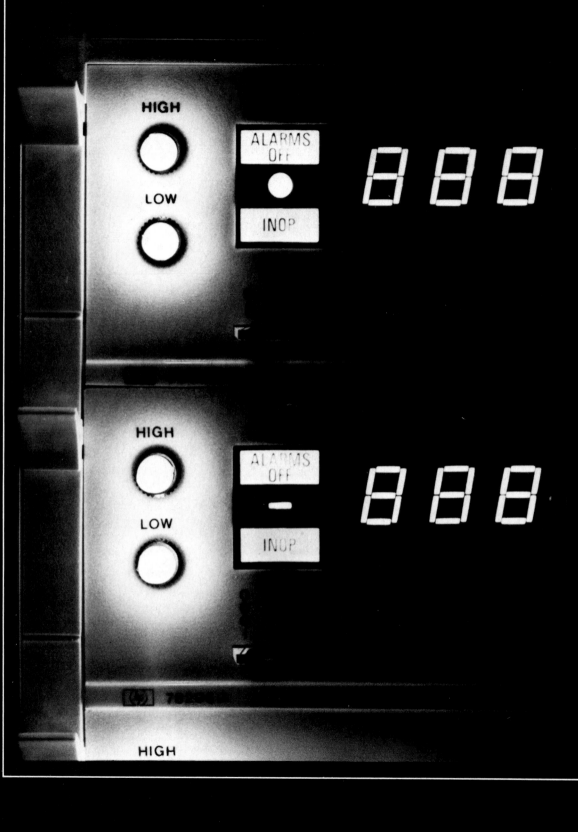

Measuring Respiratory Functions

Mass spectrometry

Apnea monitors

Transcutaneous pO₂ monitor

Mass spectrometry

Have you ever heard of a mass spectrometer? Ever *used* one? For a quick and accurate analysis of your patient's inspired and expired respiratory gases, nothing surpasses it. Moreover, you can connect the mass spectrometer to one patient or to many.

Interested in learning how the spectrometer works? How to initiate mass spectrometry? What mass spectrometry printouts look like and how to interpret them? Then read the following pages.

Why use mass spectrometry?

You can use a mass spectrometer to measure your patient's:
• respiratory rate
• inspired oxygen and carbon dioxide percentages
• expired oxygen and carbon dioxide tensions.

Since a computer controls the mass spectrometer, you can also program the monitor to calculate and display the inspiratory to expiratory ratio, the arterial-alveolar carbon dioxide gradient (a-A gradient), and other more sophisticated functions.

But mass spectrometry doesn't replace conventional blood gas measuring techniques. You'll still have to draw arterial blood to learn about arterial blood components. However, mass spectrometry can minimize the number of times you have to draw arterial blood, which saves you time and lessens patient discomfort.

Consider mass spectrometry an early-warning system. The mass spectrometer is used most often when a patient's being weaned off a ventilator. It can supply immediate data on whether or not your patient is breathing effectively on his own. Perhaps your patient's frightened, and asks to be placed on the ventilator again even though his condition doesn't warrant it. The mass spectrometer provides you with a true picture of how he's doing. Tell him about your findings, and suggest he remain off the ventilator a little longer. Then, use the mass spectrometer to monitor his expired respiratory gases continuously. Periodically, draw arterial blood samples, and send them to the lab to learn more.

Or, suppose during weaning, your patient's not exhaling the proper amount of CO_2. By using the mass spectrometer you'll find he still needs mechanical ventilation long before he exhibits signs of hypoventilation.

You can also use the mass spectrometer to monitor the effectiveness of your ventilation therapy. Is enough oxygen being delivered to your patient to maintain his blood gases at a satisfactory level? Is the positive end expiratory pressure (PEEP) you're delivering aiding your patient's CO_2 exchange effectively, or should the doctor change the PEEP setting? Is your patient's frequency of respiration set at the proper level, or is he exhaling too much or too little CO_2? These questions and more can be answered by using a mass spectrometer. In current respiratory therapy, nothing works better.

How mass spectrometry works

Have you heard of mass spectrometry? Do you know how this computer-controlled monitor can be connected to several patients at once and can analyze each one's respiratory gases? This illustration will help you understand how it works.

First, you'll place a small polyvinyl-chloride capillary tube in or near your patient's nose, or in the side port of his artificial airway. This tube, and others like it, are plugged into special wall outlets. These outlets are connected to the manifold, a unit separate from the mass spectrometer console. The manifold is maintained at a negative pressure with calibrating gas (50% O_2, 45% N_2, 5% CO_2). This pressure level helps the manifold in its sole function to traffic which patient's inhaled and exhaled air should be fed into the mass spectrometer. You simply flip a switch to instruct the manifold in its work. Then, a vacuum pump in the mass spectrometer draws the air sample from the manifold. After the gas molecules are in the mass spectrometer, they enter an ionization chamber, which first separates them by molecular weight, and then projects them onto material capable of measuring them. Finally, the mass spectrometer translates this information into either percentages of gases present or partial pressure of gases in mm Hg. This data is then displayed on the console screen and on printouts. You can have the information processed like this:
• Spot check: an immediate analysis of the respiratory gas composition of your patient's breath (printed in capnogram form).
• Trend recording: a periodic analysis of the respiratory gas composition of your patient's breaths over an extended period of time (printed in columnar form).

The mass spectrometer is more technical than most of the equipment you handle. But right now, you'll only be responsible for proper placement and maintenance of the tube. To find out more, read the following pages.

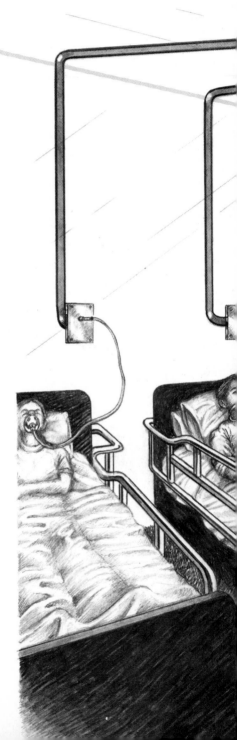

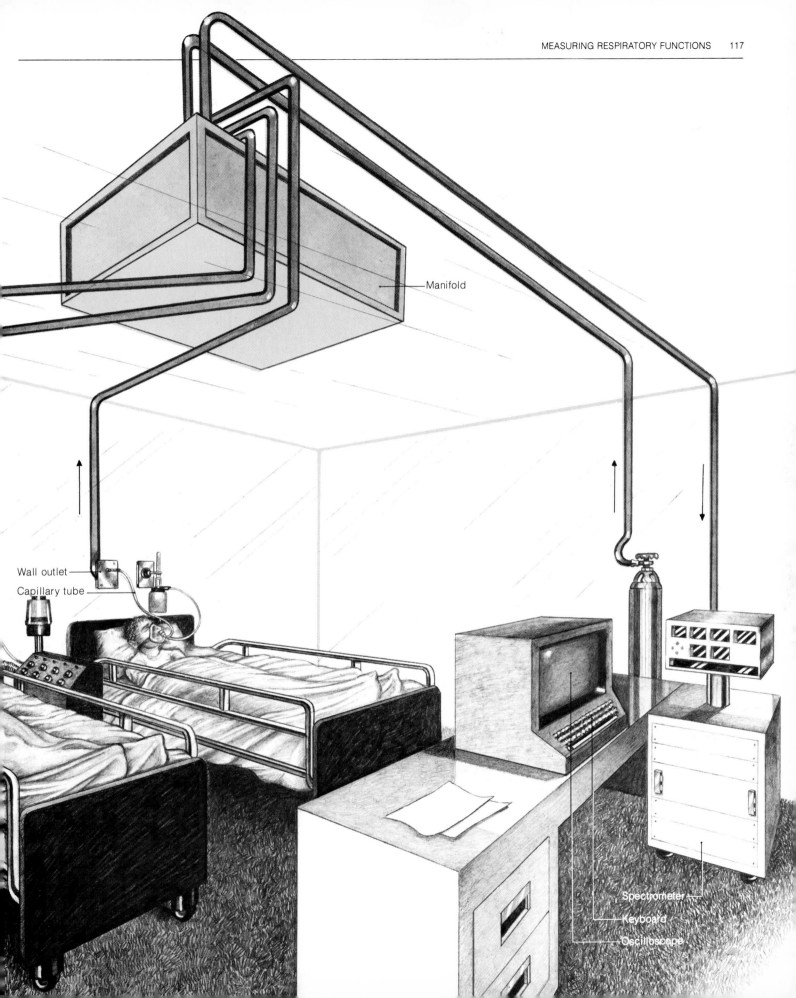

Manifold

Wall outlet

Capillary tube

Spectrometer

Keyboard

Oscilloscope

Mass spectrometry

Connecting your patient to a mass spectrometer

1 *If the doctor wants to monitor your patient's expired carbon dioxide level, he'll ask you to put the patient on a mass spectrometer. Do you know how? This photostory shows you.*

Suppose the mass spectrometry system is built into the unit at your hospital. All you'll need is a polyvinylchloride capillary tube and perhaps a rubber cork or nasal catheter. There are two types of capillary tubes: The one shown to the near right is equipped with a butterfly needle (used with the patient on a ventilator); the other one to the far right, is equipped with a blunt, malleable, 2" needle (used with the patient who isn't on a ventilator). Here's how the tube should be placed:

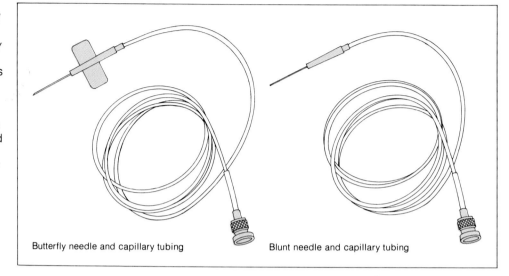

Butterfly needle and capillary tubing

Blunt needle and capillary tubing

2 For the ventilated patient with an endotracheal or tracheostomy tube in place, you'll need a capillary tube equipped with a butterfly needle and a rubber cork. Insert the butterfly needle into the cork. Make sure the needle tip goes through the other side of the cork. Then, place the cork in the side port of the swivel bar or T-piece. *Important:* Take special care never to jostle the needle or tubing. Otherwise, the needle tip may break off and be aspirated by the patient.

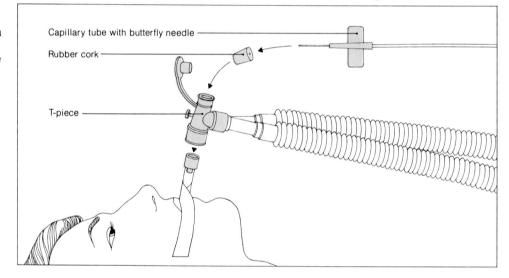

Capillary tube with butterfly needle

Rubber cork

T-piece

3 Maybe your patient isn't being mechanically ventilated but has a nasal cannula or nasal catheter in place. Then, use the capillary tube equipped with a blunt needle, and a new nasal catheter. Insert the capillary tube into the new nasal catheter. This protects the inside of the patient's nose and minimizes the risk of capillary tube occlusion. Insert the nasal catheter into one of the patient's nostrils. Ease the tube up the patient's nostril until the tube's tip lies between his naso- and oropharynx and can be seen when he opens his mouth.

☎ *Nursing tip:* If your patient is restless, you may want to secure the nasal catheter with tape.

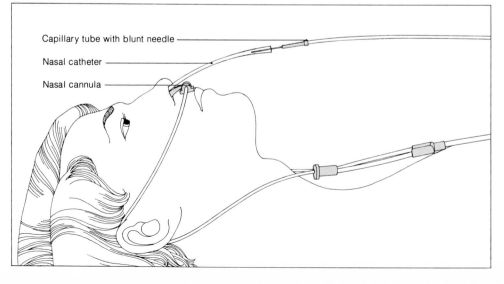

Capillary tube with blunt needle

Nasal catheter

Nasal cannula

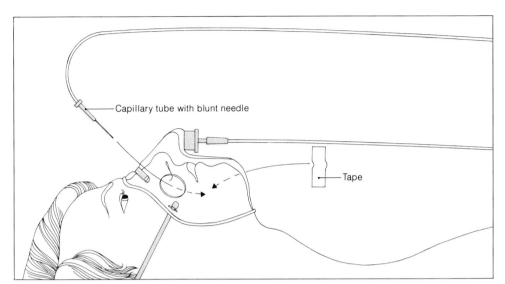

4 Perhaps your patient's receiving oxygen through a face mask. Then, insert the capillary tube equipped with a blunt needle into the hole at the side of his face mask. Secure it with tape.

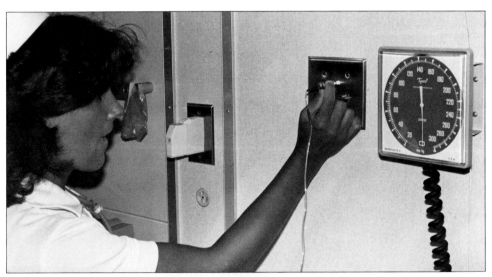

5 When the capillary tube's in place, plug the other end into the conduit outlet in the wall. If the mass spectrometer's at the patient's bedside, plug the capillary tube directly into the vacuum pump inlet.

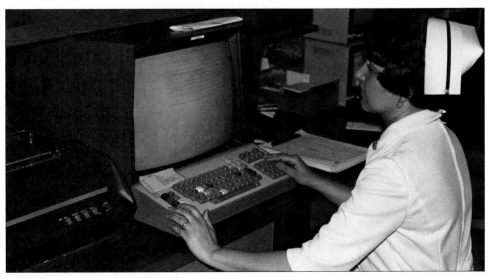

6 Then, if you've been taught how to operate the machine, enter the code required to admit a new patient to the mass spectrometry computer system. Follow this with the code that permits the spectrometer to read your patient's expiratory gas values. Finally, enter the code of the desired monitoring mode: spot check or trend recording. (For details, see the following pages.)

Important: Don't change the position of the tube if readings have already been taken. Maintaining uniform placement is crucial if you want a consistent analysis of your patient's respiratory gases.

Mass spectrometry

How to troubleshoot mass spectrometry equipment

Observation	Possible causes	Nursing action
Increase or decrease in PACO2	● Capillary tube clogged with secretions	● Replace capillary tube. ● Suction patient frequently. ● Keep patient adequately hydrated so secretions don't clog the tube.
	● Hypoventilation or hyperventilation	● Check patient's respiratory rate. Adjust ventilator, if necessary.
	● Atelectasis	● Auscultate patient frequently. Turn and sigh him hourly.
Fractional inspired oxygen (FIO2) at incorrect level	● Wrong O2 concentration	● Use an oxygen analyzer to confirm that ventilator's working properly.
	● Malfunctioning mass spectrometer	● Sample room air to confirm that mass spectrometer's working properly.
	● Condensation accumulation in ventilator tubing	● Empty condensation accumulation from ventilator tubing hourly.
LINE BLOCK alarm sounds on mass spectrometer console	● Capillary tube compressed	● Periodically make sure patient isn't lying on tubing.
	● Capillary tube clogged with secretions	● Replace capillary tube. ● Suction patient frequently.
No PACO2 waveform on oscilloscope	● Capillary tube dislodged	● Periodically check capillary tube connection and tighten, if necessary.
	● Tube disconnected from bedside or central unit	● Periodically check connection and correct, if necessary.
	● Leak in system	● Replace capillary tube.

Common printout abbreviations

To correctly interpret a mass spectrometer printout, learn the meaning of the following abbreviations:

F Resp (or Fr): The frequency of respirations means the same thing as your patient's rate of respiration for 1 minute. (The average rate is about 12 respirations per minute.)

FIO2: The fractional inspired oxygen reading tells you what percentage of the patient's inhaled air is oxygen. (The percentage of oxygen in room air is about 21%.)

FAO2: The fractional alveolar oxygen reading tells you what amount of the patient's exhaled air is oxygen. (The amount of exhaled oxygen in the breath of a patient on room air is 104 to 106 mm Hg.)

PACO2m: The partial alveolar carbon dioxide mean is the average amount of carbon dioxide—measured in millimeters of mercury—that your patient exhales with each breath in a 1-minute period. (For a healthy patient at rest, that amount falls between 38 and 44 mm Hg.)

PACO2e: The partial alveolar carbon dioxide expired reading is the greatest amount of carbon dioxide—measured in millimeters of mercury—that the patient exhales over a 1-minute period. (For a healthy patient at rest, that amount falls between 38 and 44 mm Hg.)

FICO2: The fractional inspired carbon dioxide reading tells you what percentage of the patient's inhaled air is carbon dioxide. (The percentage of carbon dioxide that the patient inhales from room air is 0.03%.)

a-A gradient: The arterial-alveolar gradient is the computerized correlation of the amount of carbon dioxide in the blood to the amount of carbon dioxide exhaled.

N: The number of readings taken (for trend recording).

CV: The coefficient variation tells you the degree of deviation between readings (for trend recording).

Reading a spot check capnogram

When you're making a spot check of your patient's respiratory function, you'll get a waveform on the mass spectrometer screen and on the printout called a capnogram. This capnogram graphically represents the amount of carbon dioxide (CO2) in each of your patient's expirations. A normal capnogram looks like this:

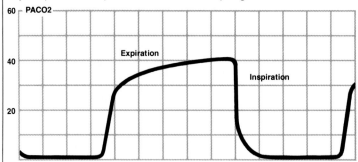

The air at the beginning of each respiration comes from the respiratory tract dead space (the trachea and bronchi), where no CO2 exchange takes place. The capnogram reflects this by registering very little CO2 at the beginning of each waveform. As a mixture of dead space air and alveolar air is expelled, CO2 content increases dramatically, reflected in the upward slope of the capnogram. Then, as all alveolar air is expelled, the capnogram plateaus at about 40 mm Hg. When the closing volume, or the end of alveolar CO2 release, occurs, the capnogram has peaked and expiration's completed. Then inspiration begins, dropping the capnogram down nearly to zero before expiration begins again. Normal inspiration-expiration cycles last about 5 seconds.

Reading a spot check capnogram continued

Centerville Hospital I.C.U.

7 Dec 80

Spot Rd Bed #3
23:55:49

F Resp	8.82
FIO2	.249
FAO2	.206
PACO2m	32.4
PACO2e	38.5
FICO2	.002

Bd	Hr:Min	Fr	FIO2	FAO2	PACO2m	PACO2e	FICO2
1	23;00	15.3	.208	.175	40.4	42.2	.001
1	22;00	15.7	.208	.142	41.3	42.7	.002
2	23;01	11.7	.398	.343	33.8	36.1	.002
2	22;01	11.5	.399	.340	35.8	40.3	.001
3	23;55	8.82	.249	.206	32.4	38.5	.002
3	23;02	8.88	.247	.205	33.3	39.7	.003
4	23;03	24.4	.386	.309	45.1	49.1	.001
4	22;03	23.6	.386	.314	44.5	51.5	.002

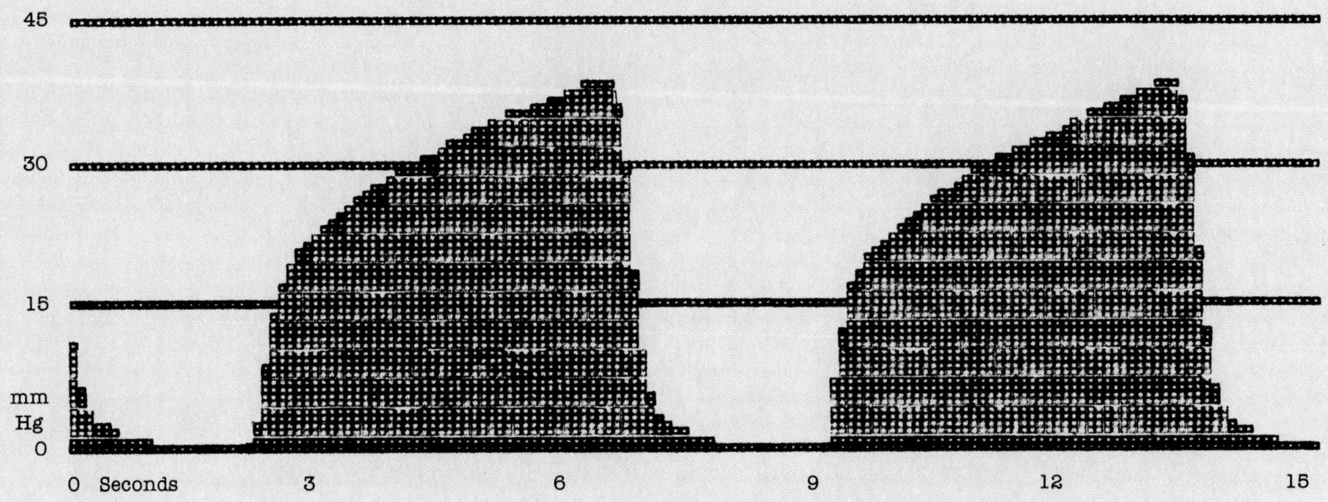

What can a capnogram tell you? Look at the example shown above. It shows the breathing pattern of a 76-year-old man with chronic obstructive pulmonary disease (COPD), postop a right middle lobectomy. If you compare this capnogram with the normal capnogram to the left, you'll see that the postop patient's waveform rises more gradually than the waveform on the other readout, and never really plateaus. This is because the closing volume occurs prematurely, gradually cutting off the alveolar CO_2 release. When you compare his expired alveolar carbon dioxide (PACO2e) peak of 38.5 mm Hg at that time with the laboratory report on his arterial carbon dioxide (PaCO2) level of 65 mm Hg, you realize he's retaining an alarmingly high amount of CO_2 (26.5 mm Hg).

While this problem is partly caused by the diseased condition of his lungs—which can't release CO_2 very effectively—it can be minimized. The doctor may increase the patient's positive end expiratory pressure (PEEP), to allow more time for CO_2 transfer from the blood to the alveoli. You should monitor the patient closely for increases or decreases in PACO2. A modest increase, which then stabilizes, is desirable. Too great an increase may indicate hyperventilation. A decrease is also undesirable, because it may indicate even greater hypoventilation and even greater CO_2 retention in the blood. For more detailed information on arterial blood gases, and PEEP, refer to the *Nursing80* PHOTOBOOK *Providing Respiratory Care*.

Mass spectrometry

Reading a trend recording

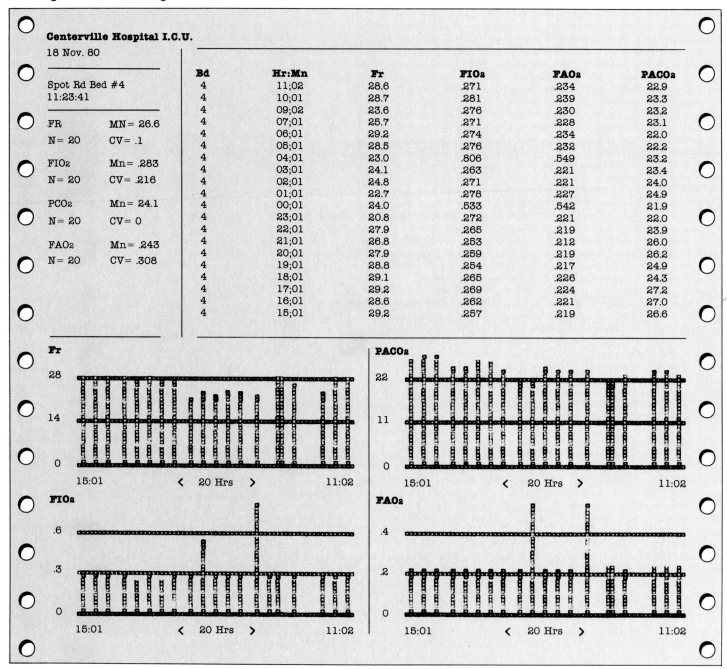

Centerville Hospital I.C.U.
18 Nov. 80

Spot Rd Bed #4
11:23:41

.FR   MN= 26.6
N= 20   CV= .1

FIO2   Mn= .283
N= 20   CV= .216

PCO2   Mn= 24.1
N= 20   CV= 0

FAO2   Mn= .243
N= 20   CV= .308

Bd	Hr:Mn	Fr	FIO2	FAO2	PACO2
4	11;02	28.6	.271	.234	22.9
4	10;01	28.7	.281	.239	23.3
4	09;02	23.6	.276	.230	23.2
4	07;01	25.7	.271	.228	23.1
4	06;01	29.2	.274	.234	22.0
4	05;01	28.5	.276	.232	22.2
4	04;01	23.0	.806	.549	23.2
4	03;01	24.1	.263	.221	23.4
4	02;01	24.8	.271	.221	24.0
4	01;01	22.7	.278	.227	24.9
4	00;01	24.0	.533	.542	21.9
4	23;01	20.8	.272	.221	22.0
4	22;01	27.9	.265	.219	23.9
4	21;01	26.8	.253	.212	26.0
4	20;01	27.9	.259	.219	26.2
4	19;01	28.8	.254	.217	24.9
4	18;01	29.1	.265	.226	24.3
4	17;01	29.2	.269	.224	27.2
4	16;01	28.6	.262	.221	27.0
4	15;01	29.2	.257	.219	26.6

Fr

28

14

0

15:01   < 20 Hrs >   11:02

PACO2

22

11

0

15:01   < 20 Hrs >   11:02

FIO2

.6

.3

0

15:01   < 20 Hrs >   11:02

FAO2

.4

.2

0

15:01   < 20 Hrs >   11:02

Suppose the mass spectrometer's been programmed to give you a trend recording. Here's what the printout can provide: as many as 21 readings of up to 11 different measurements in list form, and up to 4 different measurements in columnar form. (The doctor determines which measurements will be taken and how frequently. In this case, he has ordered 20 hourly readings of 4 measurements in list form and columnar form.)

To better understand, study this trend recording. In it, you'll see sample readings of the patient's frequency of respiration (Fr); his expired alveolar carbon dioxide (PACO2) levels; his fractional inspired oxygen (FIO2) levels; and his fractional alveolar oxygen (FAO2) levels.

As the columnar trend recording shows, the patient's Fr varies slightly. This is a common occurrence with patients like this one, who are on intermittent mandatory ventilation (IMV). The patient's PACO2 levels match the peak of each capnogram taken during the 20-hour period. Notice that his PACO2 level is basically stable, though falling slightly. This may indicate increasing CO2 retention and should be watched closely. The patient's FIO2 levels and FAO2 levels, which are being mechanically maintained, remain stable, except when he was being suctioned.

Apnea monitors

Have you ever set up and operated an apnea monitor? You'll find the task's easier than it looks. The three most crucial steps in the procedure are:
• testing the alarm system
• positioning the sensor
• setting the selector knobs.

Learn these, and you learn the basics of apnea monitoring. The following section shows you how.

Indications for apnea monitoring

An apnea monitor sounds an alarm when a patient's ventilation ceases or drops below a preset level. Apnea usually strikes the newborn, although in some instances, an older child or an adult may also be susceptible to it. Read these lists to find out the conditions that may warrant apnea monitoring.

An apnea monitor has no real substitute. Its only alternatives are around-the-clock observation or mechanical ventilation. Since around-the-clock observation is too costly for most hospitals and patients, and mechanical ventilation involves too many risks, neither alternative is practical.

Age-group
Infant/child

Conditions requiring monitoring
• Prematurity
• Neurologic disorders (for example, a congenital malformation obstructing cerebral spinal fluid [CSF] flow)
• Infant respiratory distress syndrome (hyaline membrane disease)
• Personal history of sleep-induced apnea
• Family history of sudden infant death syndrome (SIDS)

Age-group
Adult

Conditions requiring monitoring
• Neuromuscular disease (for example, Guillain-Barré syndrome)
• Narcotic or central nervous system (CNS) depressant overdose
• Inhalation of certain toxic chemicals
• Traumatic injury, not requiring mechanical ventilation
• Acute exacerbation of chronic obstructive pulmonary disease (COPD)

Understanding apnea monitors

You'll use one of two types of apnea monitors to detect respiratory problems. The more complex of the two is the impedance pneumographer. This monitor measures changes in thoracic pressure during respiration, through electrodes placed on the patient's chest in basic EKG patterns.

The other type of apnea monitor is the pressure transducer.

With this type, the transducer is placed between the patient's mattress and box spring. It detects the slight shift in the center of gravity that occurs during normal respiration.

Regardless of which type monitor you use, each one sounds an alarm when a period of apnea occurs. And both share most of the basic features, as these photos show.

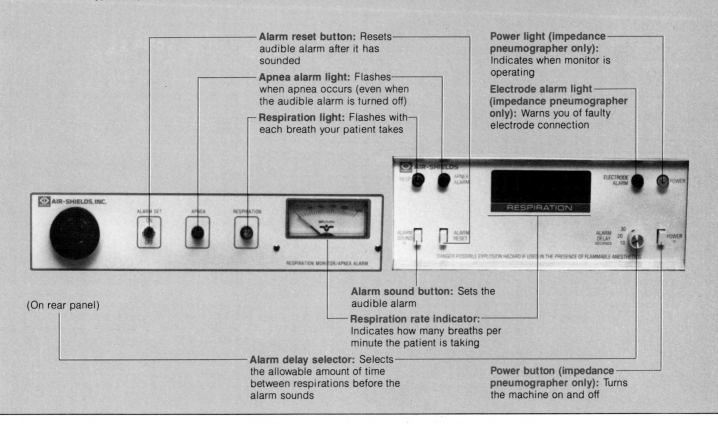

Alarm reset button: Resets audible alarm after it has sounded

Apnea alarm light: Flashes when apnea occurs (even when the audible alarm is turned off)

Respiration light: Flashes with each breath your patient takes

Power light (impedance pneumographer only): Indicates when monitor is operating

Electrode alarm light (impedance pneumographer only): Warns you of faulty electrode connection

(On rear panel)

Alarm sound button: Sets the audible alarm

Respiration rate indicator: Indicates how many breaths per minute the patient is taking

Alarm delay selector: Selects the allowable amount of time between respirations before the alarm sounds

Power button (impedance pneumographer only): Turns the machine on and off

Apnea monitors

Initiating impedance pneumography

1 *You're caring for a newborn suffering from acute drug withdrawal, and the doctor orders apnea monitoring. Do you know how to set the monitor up and use it? If not, study this photostory. We'll show you how to set up and use the most common apnea monitor, the impedance pneumographer.*

Begin by assembling the necessary equipment: the monitor, a lead wire receptor and cable, two lead wires and two electrodes (the number may vary, depending on the monitor you use), sterile gauze pad, and alcohol swabs.

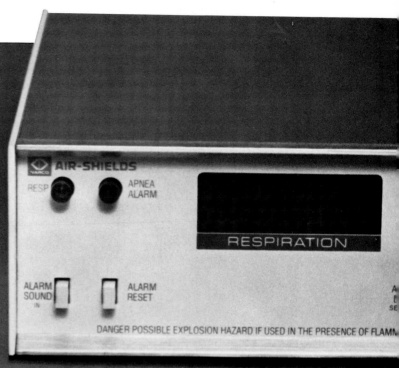

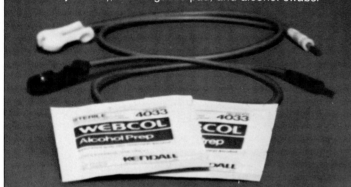

2 Remember to talk to the infant and cuddle him before you proceed. Don't assume infants are too young to require patient preparation.

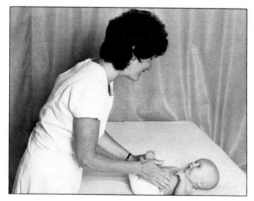

3 Now, apply an electrode to each side of the infant's abdomen, just below his rib cage, following the application procedure on pages 52 and 53.

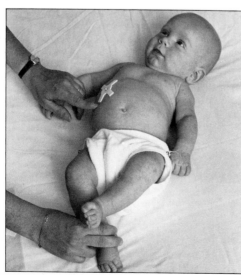

4 Connect the lead wires to the electrodes, using the manufacturer's color code.

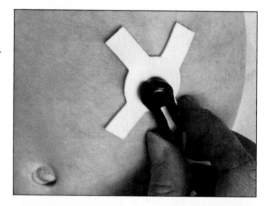

5 Attach the two lead wires to the lead wire receptor, matching the lead wires with their color-coded mates.

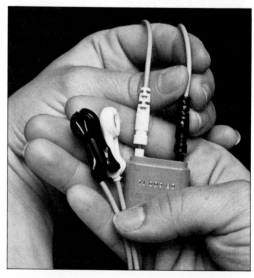

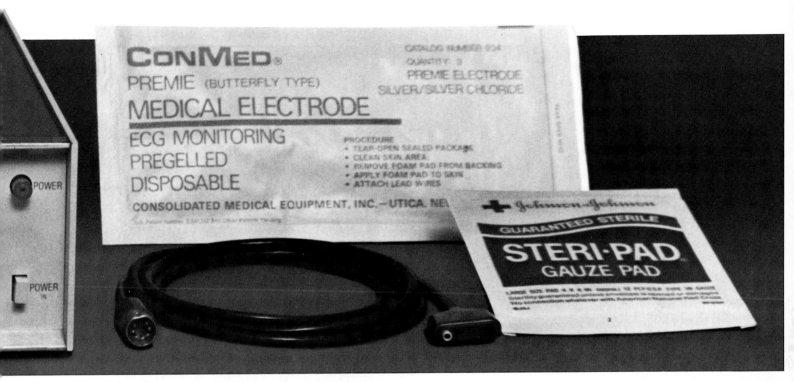

6 Plug the lead wire cable into the outlet labeled PATIENT CABLE, on the back of the monitor.

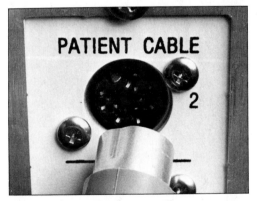

7 If the monitor isn't already plugged into a wall outlet, do so now. Make sure the electrical cable is plugged into the back of the monitor and turned slightly to the right.

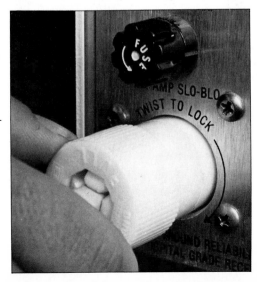

8 Depress the POWER button on the face of the monitor, as the nurse is doing here. This turns on the monitor.

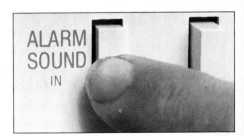

9 Then, push the ALARM SOUND button. To test the alarm, disconnect the lead wire cable from the monitor. If the alarm doesn't sound, get another monitor. If the alarm does sound, reconnect the lead wire cable, and reset the alarm.

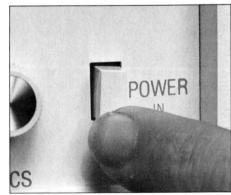

10 Finally, set the ALARM DELAY selector at 10, 20, or 30 seconds. This means the alarm will sound if the patient doesn't breathe within the time you've set. In many monitors, this setting takes the place of high and low alarms, since the main concern is the time *between* breaths, not the number of breaths per minute.

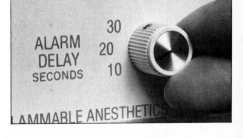

Apnea monitors

Initiating apnea monitoring with a pressure transducer

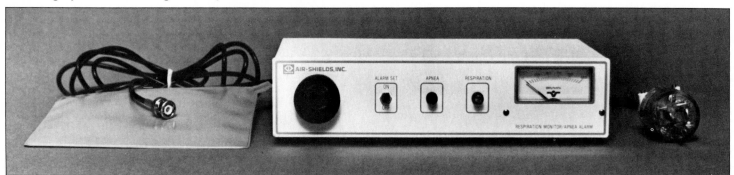

1 *If you're using a pressure transducer, sometimes called a sensor pad, for apnea monitoring, you'll find the procedure differs from that used with impedance pneumography. Using a pressure transducer is easier but not as reliable, since nothing's attached* directly to the infant.

To use a pressure transducer, follow these instructions. Begin by assembling your equipment: a pressure transducer monitor, and a pressure transducer pad.

2 Then, plug the monitor into a wall outlet. Plug the cable of the pressure transducer pad into the monitor, as shown here. To make sure the pad's working, touch it. Expect the respiration light on the monitor to blink.

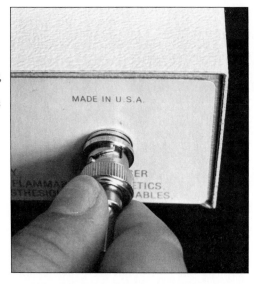

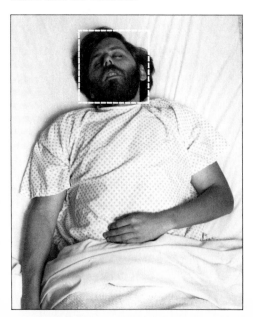

4 If you're monitoring an infant, place the pad under the mattress beneath the infant's shoulders, as this photo shows. However, for an especially active infant, it's better to place the pad beneath his midsection.

In either case, if you have difficulty obtaining a signal, get a foam rubber pad, and place the transducer pad between the foam rubber and the mattress.

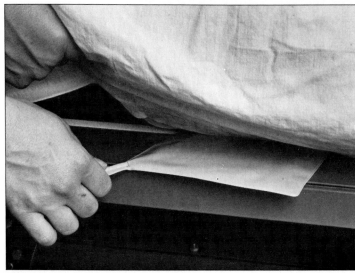

3 Place the pressure transducer pad between your patient's mattress and bed frame or box spring.

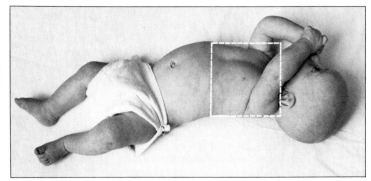

5 If your patient's an adult, place the pressure transducer pad under the mattress, just beneath his head or slightly above it. *Remember:* Regardless of where you place the pad, it must be between two flat surfaces.

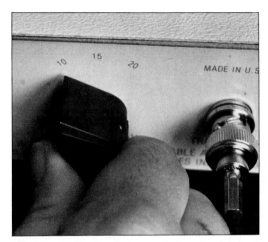

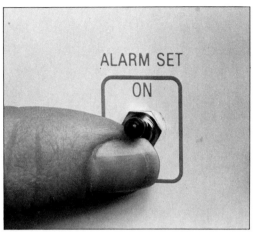

6 Locate the ALARM DELAY dial on the back of the monitoring device, and set it to the desired rate. If you set the delay dial on 10 seconds, and the infant fails to breathe in a 10-second period, the alarm will sound. If you set the delay dial on 15 seconds, the alarm will sound after 10 seconds if the infant fails to breathe, but will automatically shut off if he breathes in the next 5 seconds.

7 Finally, turn on the ALARM SET. This combination switch turns on the alarm and the monitor at the same time. Now, the monitor's counting every breath the infant takes. You'll be alerted if apnea occurs.

Going home with an apnea monitor: What to teach the parents

An infant in your care has periods of apnea. The doctor has ordered that he be sent home with an apnea monitor. You'll have to teach the infant's parents to operate it. But first, try establishing a rapport with them. If they don't trust you or won't listen to you, the teaching process will be a waste of time.

Obviously, part of your job is teaching them to operate the monitor and what's required of them when the alarm goes off. Go over the entire procedure with them several times, using the home care aid on the following pages as a guide. Give them a copy of the home care aid for their own reference. While they should know mouth-to-mouth resuscitation techniques and cardiopulmonary resuscitation (CPR), assure them that, in most cases, they'll be able to revive the child with a slight nudge. The National Sudden Infant Death Syndrome (SIDS) Foundation has produced a helpful guide to operating an apnea monitor called *A Manual for Home Monitoring.* Request it by writing to The National SIDS Foundation, 310 S. Michigan Ave., Chicago, Ill. 60604.

Counseling the parents is equally important. After they learn to operate the monitor, they must learn to accept it. But the process of adjusting to a monitor in the home may take weeks. Prepare the parents for the adjustment period by exploring some of its psychologic aspects with them. Tell them many parents don't trust the monitor at first. Fearing for their baby's well-being, they run themselves ragged. Then, with experience, they gradually realize the monitor is working for them and begin to rely on it.

Parents must never forget that their health and well-being are important, too. They may have other children to care for.

To help parents find ways to accommodate the monitor without becoming slaves to it, order the excellent booklet called *At Home with a Monitor.* It's also available through the National SIDS Foundation at the address mentioned above.

Troubleshooting apnea monitors

Problem	Possible cause and solution	Prevention
Alarm fails to sound even though the patient's respiratory rate falls below set limits	• Alarm may be malfunctioning • If your monitor has a SENSITIVITY knob, it may be set too low. Increase the setting until the alarm sounds. If the alarm still fails to sound, request monitor service.	• Test the alarm before you begin monitoring. If your monitor has a SENSITIVITY knob, set it to the proper level before you begin monitoring.
Alarm sounds intermittently even though the patient is breathing adequately	• Electrode's malfunctioning. Check the electrode for proper placement. Replace it, if necessary. • If your monitor has a SENSITIVITY knob, it may be set too high. Adjust setting.	• Make sure your equipment works before you begin. Check it at least once each shift.
Monitor displays no reading or an inaccurate one	• Electrodes or pressure transducer may be incorrectly placed. Reposition them, if necessary.	• Take special care to initiate monitoring correctly. Test all equipment first. Check cable to make sure it fits snugly in the monitor outlet.

Patient teaching

Home care

When your baby has an apnea monitor

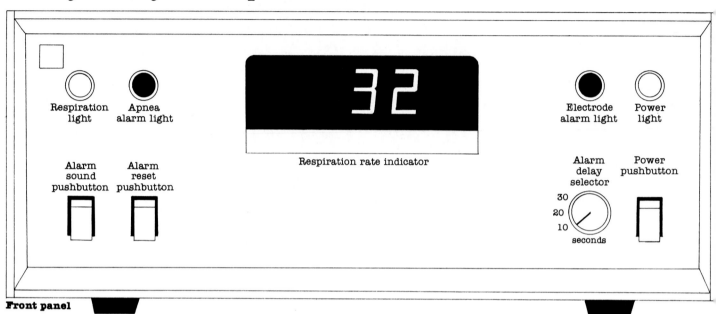

Respiration light

Apnea alarm light

Alarm sound pushbutton

Alarm reset pushbutton

Respiration rate indicator

Electrode alarm light

Power light

Alarm delay selector

30
20
10
seconds

Power pushbutton

Front panel

Dear Parents:
Your doctor and the nurses have explained why your baby needs an apnea monitor. They've also shown you how the monitor works. This home care aid will remind you of the basics.

Here are illustrations of the front and back panels of the apnea monitor you'll be taking home. If you have any questions while you're setting up the monitor about what each feature is for, refer back to this page.

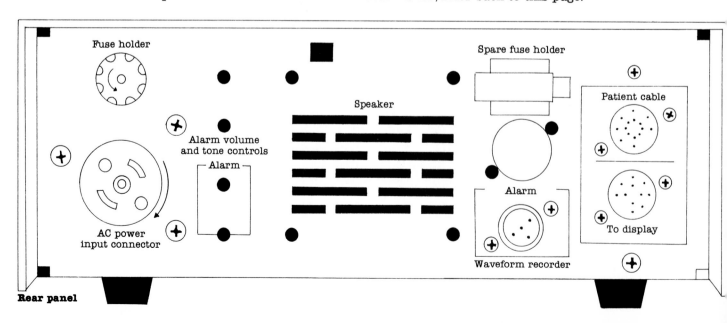

Fuse holder

Spare fuse holder

Speaker

Patient cable

Alarm volume and tone controls

Alarm

Alarm

AC power input connector

Waveform recorder

To display

Rear panel

1 Your first step in setting up the monitor is, of course, to plug it into a wall outlet. Turn it on by pressing the POWER button. When you do, expect the alarm to sound, because nothing's hooked up to the monitor.

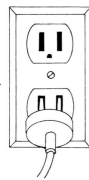

2 Turn the monitor off. Then, set the alarm delay to _____ seconds (the number ordered by your doctor).

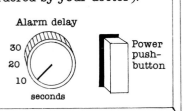

3 Plug the electrode cable into the monitor, as shown here.

4 Next, attach the lead wires to the cable.

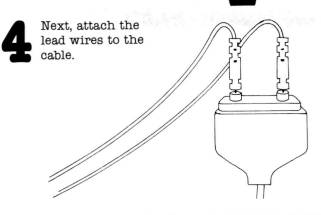

5 Then, peel the paper backing off each electrode. Apply the electrodes on both sides of your baby's chest, below his rib cage.

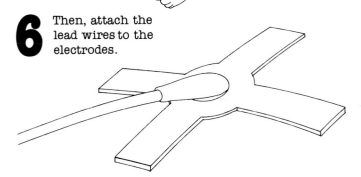

6 Then, attach the lead wires to the electrodes.

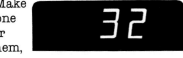

7 Turn on the monitor and watch the RESPIRATION INDICATOR. (It should light up each time your baby breathes. If it doesn't, try moving the electrodes slightly until it does.)

During the period your baby is being monitored, review basic life-support techniques occasionally. Make sure that anyone caring for your baby knows them, too.

8 Finally, keep the phone numbers of the following people handy:
• Your doctor
• Supplier of new electrodes
• Monitor repairman

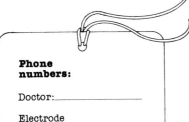

Transcutaneous pO₂ monitor

You're caring for an acutely ill infant who requires frequent checks of arterial blood gas (ABG) measurements. Which do you dislike most: Doing frequent arterial sticks or waiting for ABG determinations?

Now you can avoid both of these problems with a new noninvasive, transcutaneous blood oxygen tension monitor called the Narco Air-Shields® transcutaneous pO₂ monitor. This way of monitoring TcpO₂ is painless for the patient, simple to operate, and easy to read. To learn more about this advanced monitor, read on.

Understanding transcutaneous pO2 monitors

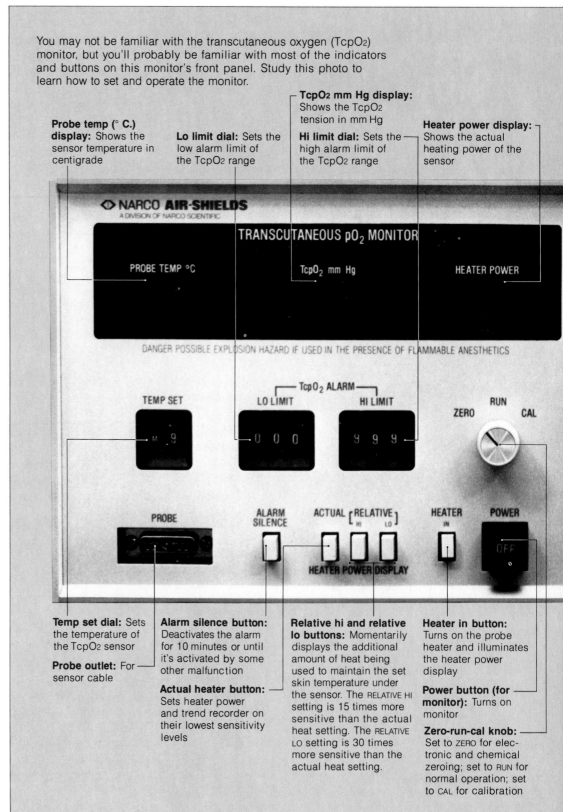

You may not be familiar with the transcutaneous oxygen (TcpO₂) monitor, but you'll probably be familiar with most of the indicators and buttons on this monitor's front panel. Study this photo to learn how to set and operate the monitor.

Probe temp (° C.) display: Shows the sensor temperature in centigrade

Lo limit dial: Sets the low alarm limit of the TcpO₂ range

TcpO2 mm Hg display: Shows the TcpO₂ tension in mm Hg

Hi limit dial: Sets the high alarm limit of the TcpO₂ range

Heater power display: Shows the actual heating power of the sensor

Temp set dial: Sets the temperature of the TcpO₂ sensor

Probe outlet: For sensor cable

Alarm silence button: Deactivates the alarm for 10 minutes or until it's activated by some other malfunction

Actual heater button: Sets heater power and trend recorder on their lowest sensitivity levels

Relative hi and relative lo buttons: Momentarily displays the additional amount of heat being used to maintain the set skin temperature under the sensor. The RELATIVE HI setting is 15 times more sensitive than the actual heat setting. The RELATIVE LO setting is 30 times more sensitive than the actual heat setting.

Heater in button: Turns on the probe heater and illuminates the heater power display

Power button (for monitor): Turns on monitor

Zero-run-cal knob: Set to ZERO for electronic and chemical zeroing; set to RUN for normal operation; set to CAL for calibration

Measuring the blood's oxygen content cutaneously

As you know, oxygen carried through a patient's arteries diffuses through his body tissue and skin. In this process, some oxygen is lost; how much is largely determined by the thickness of the epidermis. Since an infant has a relatively thin epidermis, the amount of oxygen that reaches the skin surface ($TcpO_2$) correlates closely to the amount of oxygen in the blood (PaO_2). So, by applying a special sensor to an infant's skin surface, you can measure blood oxygen tensions without drawing arterial blood.

How does an oxygen sensor work? First, it warms the patient's skin to a temperature above normal, usually 111.2° F. (44° C.), causing his cutaneous vessels to dilate. This makes it possible for oxygen in the capillary beds to diffuse through the patient's epidermis to his skin surface, where the highest level of oxygen is measured by the sensor. The illustration below shows what happens during oxygen diffusion.

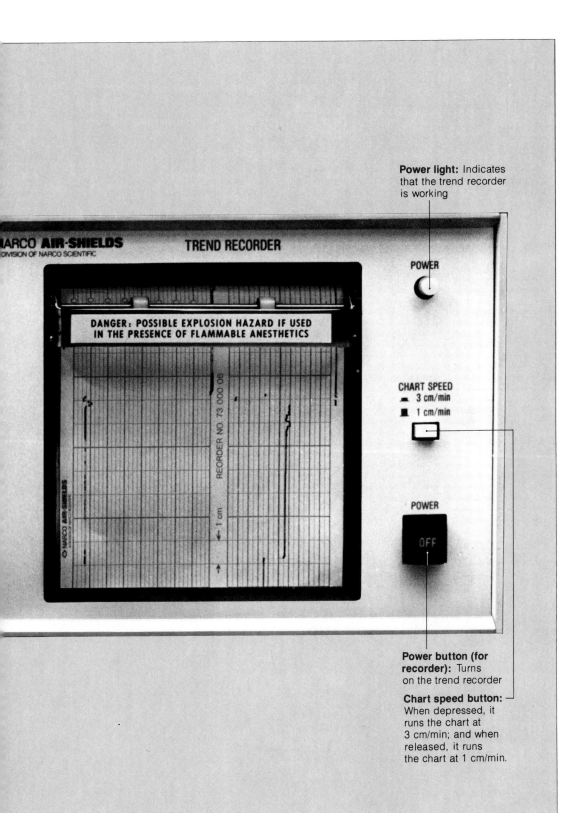

Power light: Indicates that the trend recorder is working

Power button (for recorder): Turns on the trend recorder

Chart speed button: When depressed, it runs the chart at 3 cm/min; and when released, it runs the chart at 1 cm/min.

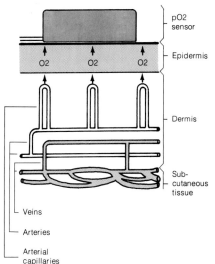

Transcutaneous pO₂ monitor

How to initiate transcutaneous pO2 (TcpO2) monitoring

1 *Setting up a TcpO2 monitor is a complex but not particularly difficult procedure if you pay attention to details and proceed slowly. This photostory shows you how it's done with a Narco Air-Shields® transcutaneous pO2 monitor.*

Begin by gathering your equipment: the TcpO2 monitor, sensor and cable, preparation block (with calibration assembly, and ejection chambers), zeroing solution, distilled water and syringe (not shown), contact jelly, adhesive ring, sterile gauze pad, and alcohol swab. If you have to replace the sensor because it has lost its sensitivity, you'll also need a new sensor membrane, electrolyte solution, and chamois cloth.

[Inset] Say a few soothing words to the infant. Then, prepare a clean, stable surface to work on.

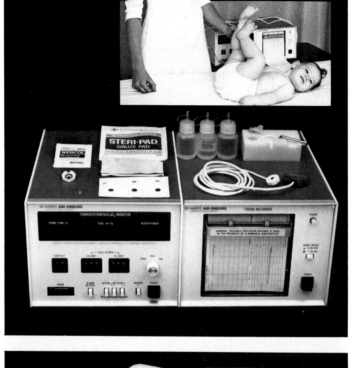

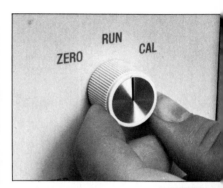

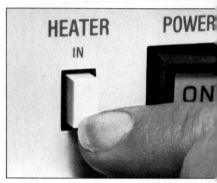

2 Now, use distilled water warmed to room temperature to fill the calibration chamber in the preparation block to the first ring.

[Inset] Place the sensor in the calibration chamber face down, and latch it in place.

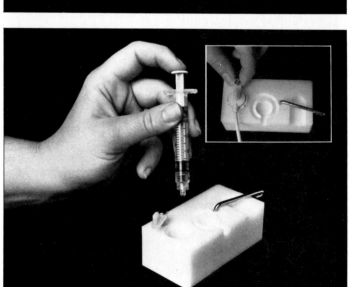

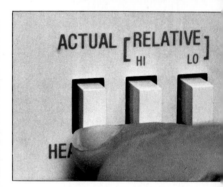

3 Make sure the monitor is turned off. Then, plug the sensor cable into the front of the monitor.

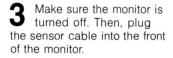

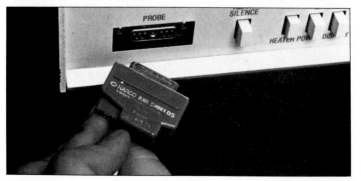

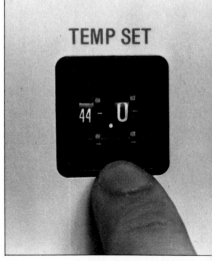

4 Turn the ZERO-RUN-CAL knob to RUN. Then, turn on the power.

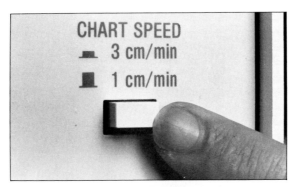

8 Turn your attention to the trend recorder side of the monitor. Depress the recorder's POWER button, and set the recorder speed at 1 CM/MIN. Expect the recorder reading to stabilize in the same manner as the mm Hg display.

5 Depress the button marked HEATER.

6 Then, depress the button marked ACTUAL HEATER, as shown here.

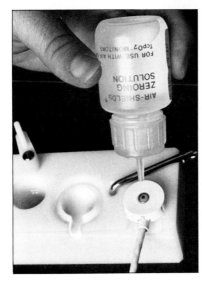

9 Now you're ready to begin chemical zeroing, which should be done once each day when the monitor's in use. To do this procedure correctly, first check the zeroing solution's expiration date. If the solution's less than a month old, use it. If it's outdated, mix up a fresh batch.

How do you prepare fresh solution? Simply empty the zeroing solution powder pack into a sterile bottle. Add the prescribed amount of distilled water. Then, immediately cap the bottle and shake it to reconstitute the powder. Label the bottle with the date the solution is prepared and the date it's due to expire (30 days later).

Now, continue the chemical zeroing procedure. Remove the sensor from the calibration chamber, and slip it face up into the assembly chamber. Place a small drop of zeroing solution over the black spot on the center of the sensor. (Recap the bottled solution immediately.) Then, observe the pO2 mm Hg display as it falls to 8 mm Hg or less within 1 minute. Make sure it's stopped falling before you proceed to the next step.

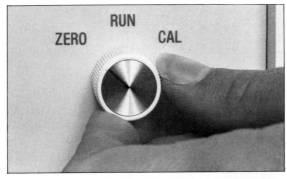

10 Now, turn the ZERO-RUN-CAL knob to ZERO. This causes the pO2 mm Hg display to register zero. Then, turn the ZERO-RUN-CAL knob back to RUN.

7 Use the thumbwheel temperature dial to set the monitor at 111.2° F. (44° C.). Within 5 to 45 minutes, the pO2 mm Hg display will stabilize between 50 and 150 mm Hg. You'll know it's stabilized if the reading doesn't vary more than 1 mm Hg for 15 minutes. If the mm Hg display doesn't stabilize in 45 minutes, you'll have to replace the sensor membrane. To find out how, see page 136. *Note:* If you ever change the temperature setting, you must recalibrate the sensor to the monitor. See step 12 of this photostory for the recalibration procedure.

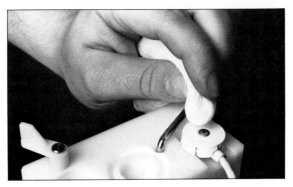

11 Use the gauze pad to wipe the zeroing solution from the sensor. Now, you've finished chemical zeroing and are ready to begin calibration.

Transcutaneous pO₂ monitor

How to initiate transcutaneous pO2 (TcpO2) monitoring continued

12 Here's how to calibrate your TcpO2 monitoring system: Place the sensor back into the calibration chamber of the preparation block, and wait for the temperature to stabilize, which'll take about 1 minute. Turn the ZERO-RUN-CAL knob to CAL.

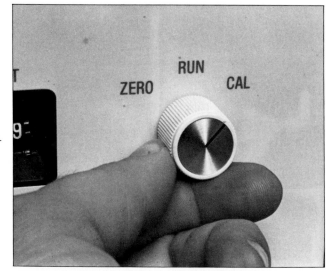

13 Watch the TcpO2 mm Hg display panel for the special calibration number that's been calculated to suit the atmospheric pressure of your local altitude. (In most areas, the number will be 154.) After that number appears, turn the ZERO-RUN-CAL knob to RUN.

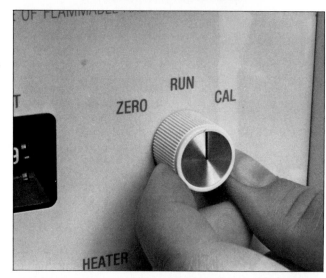

14 Take the sensor out of the calibration chamber, and slip it face up into the assembly chamber. Peel one side of the backing off the adhesive ring. Then, press that side of the ring onto the face of the sensor. Run your finger around it to seal it against the sensor face.

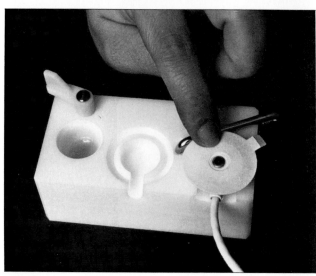

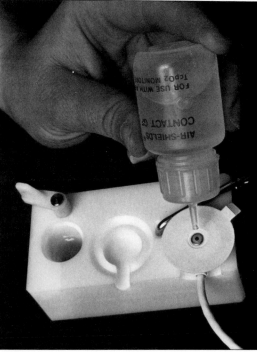

15 Place a small drop of contact jelly on the electrode portion of the sensor, being careful not to get any on the adhesive ring. However, if you do get jelly on the adhesive ring, remove the ring and replace it with a new one.

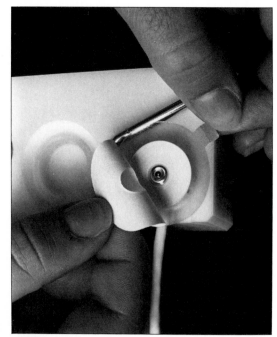

16 Peel the remaining backing from the adhesive ring. Then, use the preparation block lever to remove the sensor from the assembly chamber.

17 Clean the patient's skin around the selected site with alcohol, and let it dry.

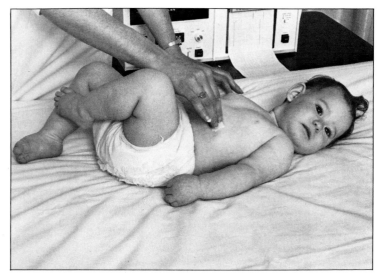

18 Place the sensor on the selected site. Press down and smooth out the adhesive ring. Run your finger around the ring to seal it. But remember, you must reposition the sensor every 3 to 4 hours or you'll irritate the patient's skin. When you do, recalibrate the sensor to the monitor, as described in step 12 of this photostory.

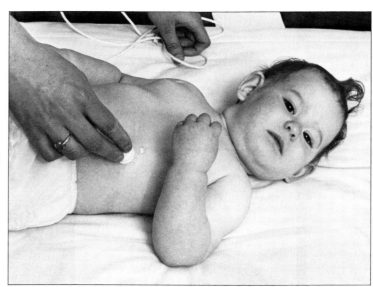

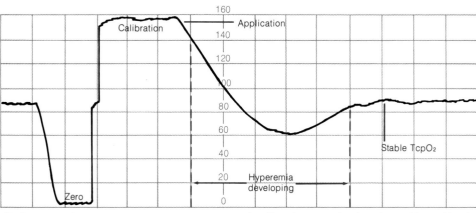

19 Immediately on application of the sensor, the recorder and pO2 mm Hg display will show a sharp drop. However, after 3 to 10 minutes, the drop will reverse itself as hyperemia develops. About 10 minutes later, the recorder and display adjust themselves and begin reflecting the patient's true TcpO2, as this waveform shows.

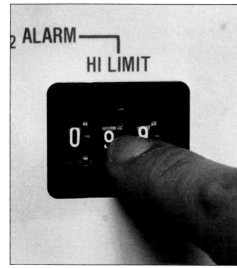

20 Set the TcpO2 LO LIMIT and HIGH LIMIT dials as ordered by the doctor. If the pO2 mm Hg display falls below the set limits, or rises above it, expect the alarm to sound.

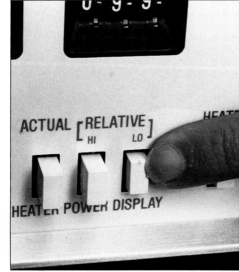

21 After 10 minutes, depress either the RELATIVE HI or the RELATIVE LO HEATER POWER DISPLAY button, depending on your patient's oxygen perfusion. This allows the monitor to display relative power changes (that is, perfusion changes). If no changes exist, the reading will be zero.

Remember to check the monitor's sensitivity daily by putting the sensor in the calibration chamber and depressing the POWER button for 5 seconds. When you turn the power on again, your pO2 mm Hg display should read between 50 and 150 mm Hg.

Transcutaneous pO₂ monitor

Replacing the sensor membrane

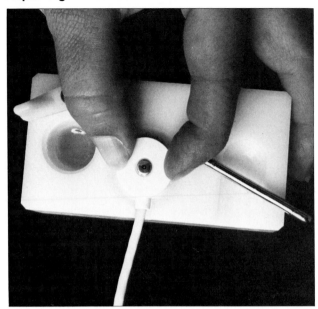

1 *What if the TcpO2 monitor reading doesn't stabilize like it should. This may indicate that something's wrong with the sensor membrane. Here's how to replace it.*

First, collect the following equipment, as shown on page 132: a new sensor membrane, preparation block, chamois cloth, sterile gauze pad, alcohol swab, and electrolyte solution. Make sure the solution isn't outdated.

Place the sensor face up into the ejection chamber of the preparation block. Using your thumb and index finger, gently press down around the face of the sensor until the membrane cap pops off. Then, discard the cap.

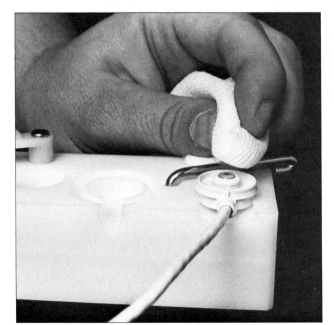

2 Lift the sensor from the ejection chamber, and place it in the assembly chamber. Use a sterile gauze pad to clean the old solution from the face of the sensor.

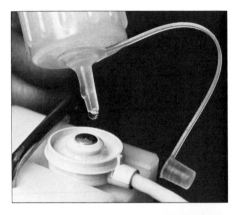

3 Place a small drop of electrolyte solution on the electrode, which is located at the center of the sensor face.

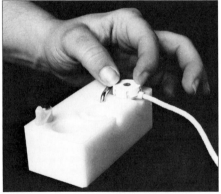

4 Using the chamois cloth, rub the surface of the electrode for about 30 seconds. Now, place another small drop of electrolyte solution on the surface of the electrode.

5 Place a new membrane cap on the sensor face. Next, press down on the rim of the cap until you hear a snap. Keep pressing around the rim until you hear six snaps. Then, the cap will be secure.

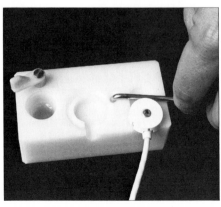

6 Now, instead of tugging on the sensor cable to remove the sensor from the assembly chamber, use the ejection lever. Examine the face of the sensor carefully. Look for wrinkles or cracks in the membrane, as well as for air bubbles in the electrolyte solution. If all's well, you'll see a clear, liquid field. If you don't, repeat the procedure. Finally, clean the face of the sensor with alcohol, and let it dry.

Troubleshooting the TcpO2 monitor

Problem	Possible causes	Nursing action
Power light doesn't light	• Unplugged monitor • Disconnected sensor cable • Defective sensor cable • Faulty wall outlet • Monitor fuse blown	• Plug monitor into wall outlet. • Secure connections at both ends of the sensor cable. • Replace sensor cable. • Use a different wall outlet. • Consult operator's manual or call for repair service.
TcpO2 mm Hg display is dark	• Monitor not warmed up yet	• Allow 10 minutes for the monitor to warm up after you turn on the power.
Trend recorder and heater power remain at zero	• Disconnected cable between TcpO2 monitor and trend recorder	• Secure cable connections.
Trend recorder chart reading doesn't agree with pO2 mm Hg display reading on monitor	• Trend recorder paper incorrectly installed	• Refer to operator's manual for proper installation technique.
Sensitivity reading is greater than 150 mm Hg	• Air bubbles on sensor face, or wrinkled or punctured sensor membrane	• Disassemble and reassemble the sensor, as described on the opposite page.
Sensitivity reading is less than 50 mm Hg but more than 8 mm Hg	• Too much electrolyte solution under sensor membrane • Leaking electrical current • Faulty sensor membrane • Deposits on sensor face	• Gently touch the membrane. If you feel a cushion of liquid, disassemble and reassemble the sensor. • Check for electrical leakage, using the procedure described in your operator's manual. • Replace membrane, using the procedure on the opposite page. • Clean sensor with an alcohol swab.
Sensitivity reading is less than 8 mm Hg	• Sensor completely disconnected • Sensor malfunctioning • Monitor malfunctioning	• Carefully reapply sensor at a different site. • Call for repair service.
TcpO2 and arterial PO2 measurements don't correlate	• Air between sensor and skin • No contact jelly on sensor • Insufficient thermal stabilization time • Sensor temperature too low • Patient has impaired arterial-alveolar perfusion or other physiologic disturbances, possibly drug induced.	• Make sure adhesive ring is tightly sealed. If not, replace it. • Remove sensor and check it. If there's no contact jelly on it, correct the problem. Then change adhesive ring and recalibrate the sensor to the monitor. • Allow 5 to 45 minutes for proper stabilization. • Increase sensor temperature. • Remove sensor and reapply it to another site. • Notify the doctor. He will order appropriate treatment.

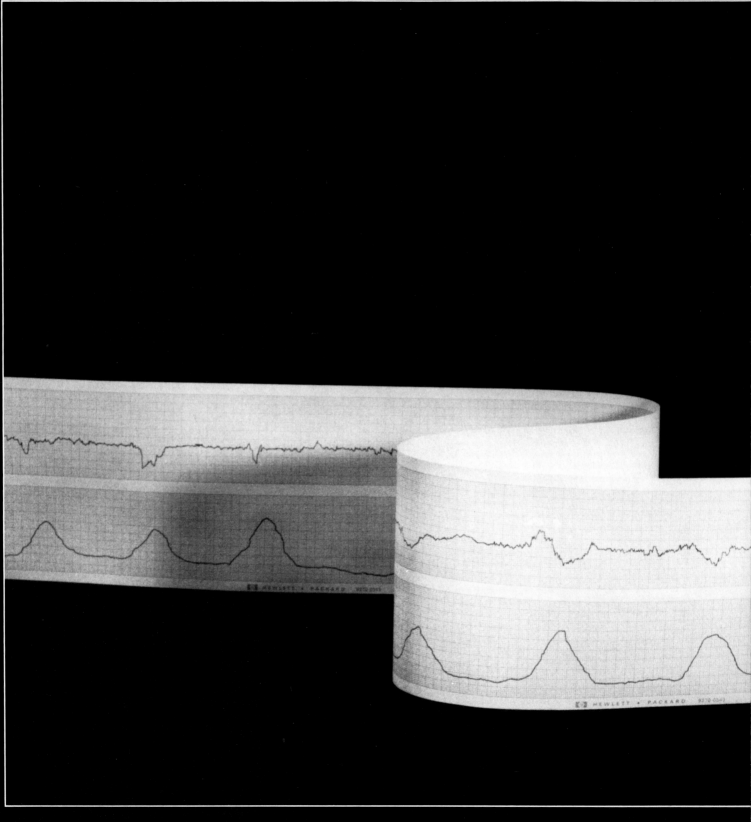

Measuring Fetal Functions

Fetal monitoring basics
External fetal monitors
Internal fetal monitors

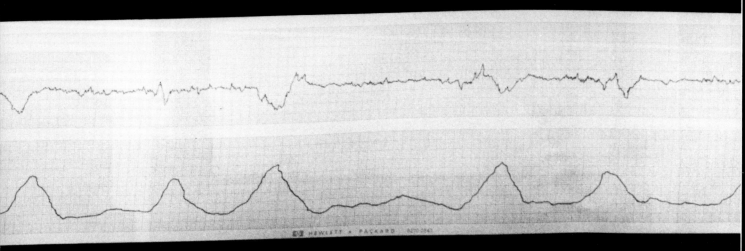

Fetal monitoring basics

In many cases, fetal monitoring is necessary for good maternal-fetal care, because it provides a way to measure maternal uterine activity, and maternal and fetal heart rate. Several types of monitors (both internal and external) are available to measure these functions. No matter which type you use, you should know how to:

• operate fetal monitors safely.
• read baseline fetal heart rate changes.
• read periodic fetal heart rate changes.
• give emotional support to the patient and her family.

The following pages will tell you how to meet these challenges. Read on to learn all you need to know about fetal monitoring.

Understanding fetal monitors

In most cases, a fetal monitor can measure several fetal functions, depending on how it's set. That's why you should become familiar with the features of the monitor before you begin any procedure. Study the one we picture here, and learn the purpose of each feature.

Oscilloscope: Displays these waveforms: fetal heart rate (FHR), maternal-fetal EKG, or fetal EKG

Freeze button: Freezes the EKG or FHR waveform on the oscilloscope screen for inspection

Test button: Produces a 120 beat per minute (bpm) pattern on the recorder paper and on the HEART RATE DISPLAY, and simulates 50 mm Hg on the uterine activity section of the recorder paper for calibration purposes

Edit/unedit switch: Selects how the signals of external monitoring modes will be processed

Maternal heart rate (MHR) button: Records maternal heart rate on the recorder paper and shows this rate on the HEART RATE DISPLAY (with abdominal EKG mode only)

Plot uterine activity (UA) button: Produces a plot display of UA units on the uterine activity section of the recorder paper

Ultrasound/direct doppler: Determines how ultrasonic signals will be processed

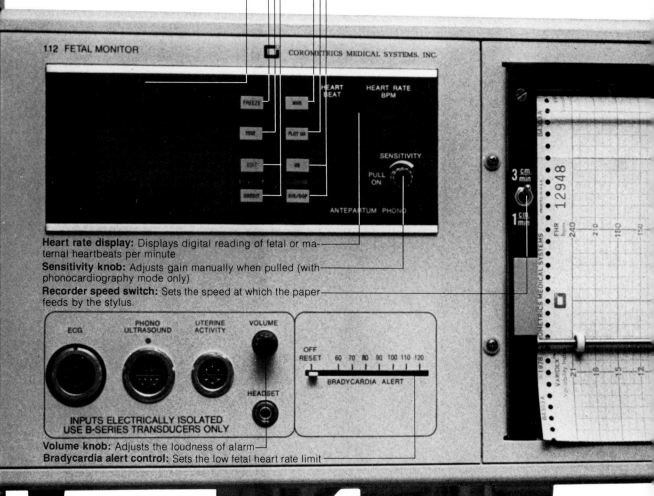

Heart rate display: Displays digital reading of fetal or maternal heartbeats per minute
Sensitivity knob: Adjusts gain manually when pulled (with phonocardiography mode only)
Recorder speed switch: Sets the speed at which the paper feeds by the stylus.

Volume knob: Adjusts the loudness of alarm
Bradycardia alert control: Sets the low fetal heart rate limit

Record button: Turns the recorder on and off

Mark button: Imprints an arrow on the uterine activity section of the recorder paper

Pressure zero indicator: Flashes when uterine pressure is less than zero

Power button: Turns monitor on and off

Printout: Records fetal heart rate on its left side and uterine activity on its right side

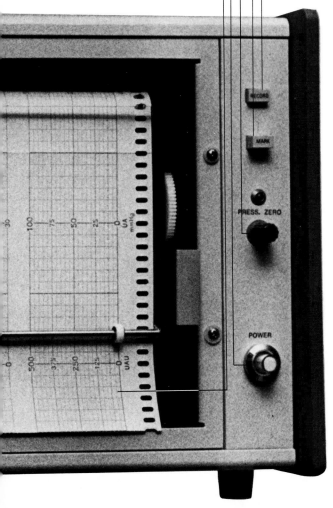

Understanding maternal-fetal physiology

Fetal health depends on unobstructed blood circulation between (and within) the fetus and the mother. As you can see in this illustration, these two circulatory systems consist of four distinct vascular systems: the uterine blood supply, the maternal intervillous space, the fetal chorionic villous in the placenta, and the fetal circulatory system.

The mother's and fetus' blood never mix. Rather, oxygen and nutrients are transferred from the mother's blood to the fetus' blood in this manner: First, maternal blood fills the intervillous space, which is interwoven with fetal chorionic villi. The thin-walled fetal capillaries in the villi (see inset) then absorb oxygen and nutrients from the mother's bloodstream. After absorption, the oxygen and nutrients enter the fetus' bloodstream.

If this transfer is jeopardized in any way, the fetus may suffer irreparable harm. Monitoring fetal functions helps identify problems before they become life-threatening.

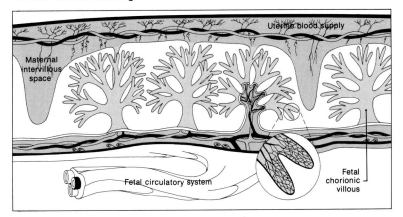

PATIENT PREPARATION

Preparing the patient

What's the first thing a pregnant woman thinks of when she sees a fetal monitor? She probably thinks that something's wrong with her baby. Never assume she knows *all* she should know about fetal monitors, even if she's been fortunate enough to attend childbirth education classes. Instead, find out what she does know *before* you bring the monitor into the labor room.

Explain the monitoring procedure, as well as why she needs it. Encourage her to ask questions, and try to answer them completely. Correct any misconceptions she may have. Stress that the monitor helps assess fetal well-being. Don't describe the monitor as a way to look for problems, but rather as a way to help avert them.

When you've completed these steps, bring the monitor into the labor room. But don't become so preoccupied setting up the monitor that you forget your patient. Talk to her as much as possible throughout the entire monitoring procedure.

Reassure her support persons, too. Explain monitoring to them, just as you did with your patient. Answer all their questions and, if policy permits, involve a member of the patient's family in her care.

Remember: The key to accurate monitoring is more than knowing how to operate equipment. Never forget your responsibilities to everyone involved: the fetus, the mother, and their loved ones.

Fetal monitoring basics

Nurses' guide to baseline fetal heart rate

By knowing how to interpret fetal heart rate (FHR), you can learn much about the fetus' well-being. To do this, take three basic FHR measurements: baseline rate, baseline variability, and periodic rate. This chart tells you all you need to know about baseline FHR and baseline variability. The chart to the right explains periodic rate.

To determine the baseline FHR, study a monitor printout for at least 1 minute, doing this *before* the mother goes into labor or *between* uterine contractions. Average the FHR readings for this minute. Or, you can average the FHR for 1 minute using the digital display. A normal baseline FHR ranges between 120 and 160 beats per minute (bpm).

After you've determined the baseline FHR, determine variability, which is the amount the baseline FHR varies from minute to minute. Normal variability ranges between 6 and 10 bpm.

If you detect an abnormal baseline rate or variability, suspect complications. Consult this chart to find out what to do about them.

Reading	Problem	Possible causes	Nursing intervention
Baseline beats per minute (bpm)	• Tachycardia (baseline FHR over 160 bpm)	• Mild fetal hypoxia • Fetal infection • Fetal neurologic immaturity • Maternal fever • Maternal tachycardia • Maternal anxiety • Maternal cardiac arrhythmia • Thyroid hormones given to mother during pregnancy	• Closely monitor maternal vital signs. • Change maternal position.
	• Bradycardia (baseline FHR under 120 bpm)	• Congenital fetal heart disorders • Fetal distress (when accompanied by changes in baseline variability) • Antiarrhythmic drugs given to mother during pregnancy • Maternal hypothermia • Postmature fetus	• Notify doctor immediately. • Change maternal position. • Administer oxygen to mother. • Prepare for immediate delivery.
Baseline variability	• No variability (baseline FHR does not vary from minute to minute)	• Fetal acidosis (especially if accompanied by late deceleration) • Fetal neurologic immaturity • Analgesic given to mother.	• Note time and dose of all maternal medication in nurses' notes. • See the Late deceleration entry in the chart on the opposite page.
	• Decreased variability (baseline FHR varies less than 6 bpm)	• Incomplete maturation of the fetal parasympathetic nervous system • Physiologic sleep (periodic fetal sleep cycles lasting 20 to 30 minutes) • Anesthetic or analgesic given to mother. • Fetal cardiac arrhythmias • Fetal hypoxia • Fetal acidosis • Fetal asphyxia	• Recalculate fetal age. • Stimulate fetus externally by shaking mother's abdomen, changing her position, or administering oral glucose (orange juice). • Notify doctor, if sedative effects seem excessive. Administer antidote, if ordered. • Notify doctor if you detect fetal cardiac arrhythmias.
	• Increased variability (baseline FHR varies more than 10 bpm)	• Maternal or fetal activity • Maternal hypoxia • Maternal anxiety • Analgesic given to mother. • Fetal acidosis • Fetal neurologic immaturity • Tetanic uterine contractions	• Check uterine contractions for duration and frequency. • Allow time for fetus to quiet down. Palpate abdomen to check fetal position. • Change maternal position. • Notify doctor if problem persists.

Nurses' guide to periodic fetal heart rate

What is periodic fetal heart rate (FHR) and how do you interpret it? Periodic FHR shows you how the fetal heart rate is affected by uterine contractions.

Periodic FHR reveals one of the following:
• acceleration (when the FHR increases with uterine contractions)
• deceleration (when the FHR decreases with uterine contractions).

Deceleration is further divided into early, late, and variable decelerations, depending on *when* it occurs during uterine contractions.

Study this chart. It'll tell you more about periodic fetal heart rate, including any necessary nursing interventions.

Type	Possible causes	Characteristics	Clinical significance	Nursing intervention
Acceleration	• Stimulation of the fetus' autonomic nervous system. Normal response to umbilical cord compression during uterine contraction.	• Usually 15 beats or more per minute (bpm) above the baseline rate • May occur before, during, or after a contraction • May occur with each contraction • Usually associated with average baseline variability and, occasionally, with smooth or decreased baseline variability • Compensatory accelerations may occur after variable decelerations.	• Acceleration, along with fetal movement, usually indicates fetal well-being. • Uniform accelerations occurring late during contraction are often followed by a pattern of late decelerations.	• Explain the significance of fetal heart rate (FHR) accelerations to the mother and her support person, if present.
Early deceleration	• Compression of the fetus' head	• Waveforms uniform in shape, usually a mirror image of contraction. • Usually doesn't fall below 100 bpm • Onset occurs early in the contraction. • May occur with each contraction • Usually associated with average baseline variability	• Benign and usually well tolerated by the fetus. • Not associated with uteroplacental circulatory insufficiency • Persistent, progressive decelerations without descent of the fetus and/or excessive molding of the fetus' head may indicate possibility of cephalopelvic disproportion (CPD).	• Explain the significance of early decelerations to the mother and her support person, if present. Reassure them that the fetus is well.
Late deceleration	• Uteroplacental circulatory insufficiency (placental hypoperfusion), caused by decreased intervillous blood flow during the contractile phase of labor • Uterine hyperactivity from excessive infusion of oxytocin • Maternal hypotension • Maternal supine hypotension syndrome	• Waveform is U-shaped, usually a mirror image of contraction. *Note:* Don't confuse late decelerations with early decelerations. They are similiarly shaped but occur at different times during the contraction. • May occur during one or more contractions • When associated with normal baseline variability, late decelerations usually indicate impaired transfer of oxygen and nutrients between mother and fetus. • When associated with increased variability or tachycardia and no variability, late decelerations indicate depression of fetal central nervous system and fetal myocardial hypoxia.	• Any late deceleration is considered significant; the longer it persists, the more serious it becomes. • When the problem causing late decelerations is corrected, the fetus usually recovers and labor continues. • When the problem causing late decelerations is corrected but late decelerations persist, fetus may be hypoxic and asphyxiated.	• If the cause is uteroplacental circulatory insufficiency, increase I.V. fluid rate to increase maternal cardiac output. • If the cause is uterine hyperactivity, discontinue oxytocin infusion, and time uterine contractions. • If the cause is maternal hypotension, elevate the mother's legs to increase venous return. • If the cause is maternal supine hypotension syndrome, turn the mother on her left side to relieve pressure on her inferior vena cava. • Regardless of the cause, administer oxygen to increase oxygen saturation of maternal blood. • Notify doctor. He may take a fetal capillary blood sampling to check for fetal acidosis. • Explain the significance of late decelerations and your nursing intervention to the mother and her support person, if present.
Variable deceleration	• Compression of umbilical cord, causing decreased oxygen perfusion to fetus, followed by either the collapse of the umbilical vein and fetal hypotension, or the occlusion of the umbilical arteries and fetal hypertension	• Sudden drop in FHR with irregular waveforms, usually shaped like the letter V, U, or W • Onset occurs before, during, or after a contraction. • FHR usually decelerates below 100 bpm, with a quick return to baseline. The range of deceleration may be mild, moderate, or severe. • Unpredictable rate of occurrence	• Most variable decelerations are not serious. • Severe prolonged variable decelerations are associated with fetal hypoxia, and result in baseline tachycardia and loss of baseline variability. • FHR changes usually begin 45 to 60 seconds after umbilical cord compression. • Fetus' well-being depends on frequency and duration of umbilical cord compression. • Most healthy fetuses can tolerate repeated decelerations up to 45 seconds without distress.	• Explain variable decelerations and nursing intervention to the mother and her support person, if present. • Change maternal position to relieve umbilical cord compression. • Increase I.V. fluid rate to increase maternal blood volume. • Administer oxygen to increase maternal $PaCO_2$. • If infusing oxytocin, discontinue therapy.

External fetal monitors

Some doctors routinely apply external fetal monitors on all their patients who are in labor. Others reserve external fetal monitors for high-risk patients: for example, those with a history of complications.

What can external fetal monitoring tell you? It provides quick information about rate, duration, and intensity of the patient's uterine contractions and how they're affecting the fetus' heart rate (FHR). Learn more about this method of fetal monitoring by reading this section. Then you'll be able to answer the following questions:
• How do you determine fetal position?
• When is conduction jelly used?
• Where on the patient's abdomen are the electrodes applied?
• What do you do to correct an inadequate reading?

Learning about external fetal monitors

What types of external fetal monitoring equipment does your hospital use? On the following pages, we'll show you how to use four types. To monitor uterine activity, use a tocotransducer. To monitor the fetal heart rate (FHR), use either an ultrasonic transducer or a phonotransducer. To monitor the FHR and maternal-fetal EKG, use abdominal electrodes.

Tocotransducer: This features a pressure-sensitive button which, when placed on the uterine fundus, detects uterine activity. This activity is then relayed to the monitor, which records the frequency and duration of uterine contractions. The toco-transducer is usually used in combination with an FHR monitor.

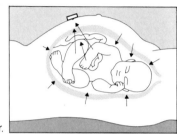

Ultrasonic transducer: This sends low-energy, high-frequency sound waves through the abdominal wall in the direction of the fetal heart. These sound waves strike the fetal heart wall and are deflected back through the abdominal wall. The ultrasonic transducer then receives the deflected

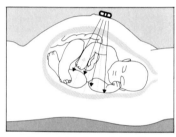

waves and relays them to the fetal monitor, which translates them into audible fetal heart tones and FHR waveforms. Because ultrasound reflects mechanical heart movement instead of actual electrical conduction, expect only an approximate heart rate, not a true one.

Phonotransducer: This detects FHR using a microphone placed on the mother's abdomen. The microphone amplifies fetal heartbeat, and the monitor translates these tones into a FHR waveform. Don't use the phonotransducer on a woman in advanced labor, because the microphone will respond to all movements and sounds, making the waveforms inaccurate.

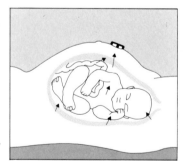

Abdominal electrodes: These are used to measure fetal and maternal heart rates. Unlike the other FHR monitoring methods, abdominal electrodes also yield a maternal-fetal EKG. The maternal-fetal EKG appears on the oscilloscope screen. The FHR waveform is printed on the printout paper.

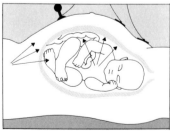

Most brands of fetal monitors can adequately distinguish between the maternal and fetal EKG to provide an accurate waveform. But you may get an inaccurate waveform if the mother or fetus moves, or the mother is obese. You may also get an inaccurate waveform if the fetus is less than 28 weeks old, because the QRS complex will be too small to measure.

Performing Leopold's maneuver

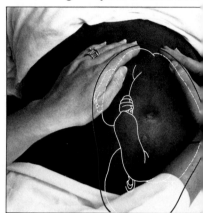

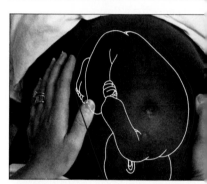

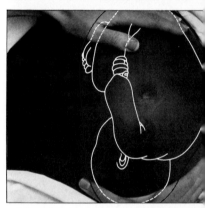

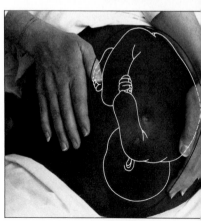

Many monitoring procedures require that you know fetal position for accurate placement of a transducer or electrodes. How can you tell? By doing the four Leopold's maneuvers, in the order shown here.

1 First maneuver: Stand over your patient, and gently place your hands on both sides of her abdomen, curling your fingers around her uterine fundus. If the fetus is in the vertex position—left occiput anterior (LOA)—you'll feel an irregularly shaped, soft object: the fetus' buttocks. If the fetus is in the breech position, you'll feel a hard, round, movable object: the fetus' head.

2 Second maneuver: Now, move your hands down the sides of your patient's abdomen, applying firm, even pressure inward. On one side you should feel a smooth, hard surface offering resistance: the fetus' back. For example, if the fetus is in the vertex position (LOA), its back will probably be facing the left side of the mother's abdomen.

On the right side of the mother's abdomen, expect to feel some irregular knobs or lumps: the fetus' hands, feet, elbows, and knees.

If the fetus is in a breech position, its back will be more difficult, if not impossible, to find.

3 Third maneuver: Next, spread apart the thumb and fingers of one hand (as wide as possible), and place them just above the mother's symphysis pubis. Bring your thumb and fingers together. If the fetus is in the vertex position (LOA) and you feel its head, you can assume it *hasn't* descended into the uterine canal. But if you feel a less distinct mass, you'll know it *has* descended. If the fetus is in the breech position and you feel its buttocks, the fetus hasn't descended. If you feel its back, then it has descended.

To determine how *far* the fetus has already descended, no matter what position it's in, do the fourth maneuver.

4 Fourth maneuver: Turn and face the mother's feet. Place your hands on both sides of her lower abdomen, at the midline. Applying gentle pressure, slide your hands downward, toward your patient's vagina. If the fetus is in the vertex position (LOA) and you feel its head, then the head isn't engaged in the pelvic inlet. But if you have trouble feeling the head, then it is probably engaged. If the fetus is in the breech position and you feel its hips, the buttocks probably aren't engaged in the pelvic inlet. If you have trouble feeling the hips, the buttocks are engaged.

Now with the completion of this maneuver, you have a fairly accurate idea of how the fetus is positioned in the mother's uterus.

Locating fetal heart beat

As you know, the fetus can be in any one of several positions in the mother's uterus. By performing Leopold's maneuvers, you can determine approximate fetal position. Here's an additional aid to help you locate the site that will yield the clearest fetal heart sounds. When you must place an external fetal monitor on the mother's abdomen to record fetal heart sounds, use this illustration as a guide.

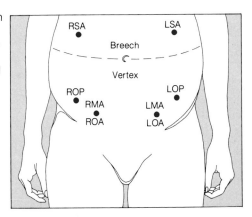

Using a tocotransducer to monitor uterine activity

Mrs. Phillips has begun labor in her fourth pregnancy. Her last pregnancy ended in a stillbirth. The two babies before were small and born prematurely. Because of this history, the doctor wants to monitor her labor carefully. You'll be monitoring both uterine activity and fetal heart rate. Here, you'll find out how to monitor uterine activity. On the next page, you'll discover various ways you can monitor fetal heart rate. For uterine activity monitoring, you'll need

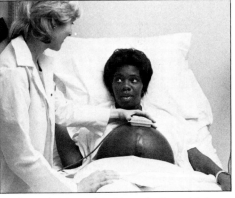

this equipment: a fetal monitor, a tocotransducer and cable, a belt, and talc.

Tell your patient what you're going to do and why. Then, follow these steps:
- Plug the tocotransducer into the monitor inlet labeled UTERINE ACTIVITY.
- Turn on the monitor and depress the printout button.
- Turn the PEN SET knob on the tocotransducer until the stylus moves to zero on the right (or uterine activity) side of the printout paper. As you've probably noticed, the printout paper is divided into two parts. On the left side, the fetal heart rate waveform is recorded. On the right side, the uterine activity waveform is recorded.
- Place the tocotransducer over the uterine fundus, which you can locate by doing the Leopold's maneuvers.
- Slip the belt under your patient.
- *Nursing tip:* Powder the belt, so it's less irritating.
- Between contractions, secure the tocotransducer with the belt, tightening the belt until the stylus on the right side of the printout paper moves to the 50 mm Hg mark. *Important:* Never do this procedure during a contraction.
- Then, turn the PEN SET knob until the stylus moves back to approximately the 10 mm Hg marking on the printout paper. At this point, the monitor is ready to record uterine activity.
- Test the tocotransducer by pressing down on it slightly. This pressure should cause the recorder baseline to waver. If it doesn't, get another pressure transducer and repeat the test. Finally, document the procedure in your nurses' notes.

Remember: External monitor readings of uterine activity tell you the frequency and duration of contractions. But because you're monitoring externally, the waveforms may also reflect your patient's coughs, retches, or position changes. Mark this type of activity on the printout paper when it occurs, so the waveforms aren't misinterpreted. (For more precise monitoring that also measures the intensity of contractions, the doctor will probably use internal uterine pressure monitoring, described on pages 152 and 153.)

External fetal monitors

Monitoring fetal heart rate (FHR)

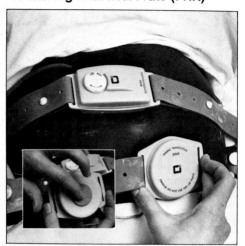

Using a phonotransducer

The doctor wants Mrs. Phillips' fetal heart rate to be monitored, as well as her uterine activity, which was discussed on the preceding page. You can use any one of three methods to detect FHR: phonocardiography, ultrasound, or abdominal electrocardiography. Here you'll find out how to use a phonotransducer. The other methods will be explained in the stories that follow.

First, gather a fetal monitor, a phonotransducer with attached cable, a belt, and talcum powder. (Note that you do not use electrode jelly with this device.) Then, follow these steps:
• Plug the phonotransducer cable into the monitor inlet marked PHONO.
• Turn on the monitor. Then, gently tap the transducer to make sure it's working properly, as shown in the inset. If it is, you'll hear a magnified audio signal of the tapping.
• Depending on the doctor's orders, choose between the EDIT and the UNEDIT button. If you press the EDIT button, the monitor will average every three heartbeats and will edit out most artifacts (waveform interference). If you press the UNEDIT button, every heartbeat is displayed on the oscilloscope screen.
• Make sure your patient's abdomen is clean and dry. Position the phonotransducer on her abdomen, and locate the clearest heartbeat sounds. If the fetus is in the vertex position—left occiput anterior (LOA)—you'll probably find the clearest

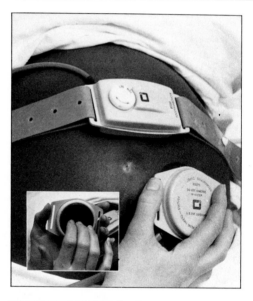

Using an ultrasonic transducer

An alternate method of FHR monitoring involves an ultrasonic transducer. Do you know how to use one? Here's how:

Begin by gathering this equipment: a fetal monitor, an ultrasonic transducer with attached cable, ultrasonic jelly, a belt, and talcum powder. Then, follow these steps:
• Plug the transducer cable into the fetal monitor inlet labeled ULTRASOUND. The doctor will decide whether to use the directional doppler (DIR/DOP), which picks up only fetal heart movement that's within a narrow range, or conventional doppler (US), which picks up all fetal heart movement. Press the appropriate button.
• Next, choose between the EDIT and the UNEDIT buttons. As you may know, the EDIT mode averages every three heartbeats and edits out distortion. The UNEDIT mode simply displays each heartbeat.
• Now, turn on the monitor. Gently tap the diaphragm of the transducer to make sure it's working properly (as shown in the inset to the left). If it is, you should hear a magnified audio signal of your tapping.
• Use the first and second Leopold's maneuvers to determine fetal position. Then, locate the site that yields the best fetal heart tones.
• Now, apply ultrasonic jelly to the transducer diaphragm. Cover the diaphragm completely to form an effective seal. If you don't, air leaks may interfere with sound waves and create inadequate waveforms.
• Position the transducer on the selected site, adjusting it as needed, to get the best fetal heart tone, as the nurse is doing in the large photo to the left. As you move the transducer, don't lose contact with the patient's skin.

How will you know the transducer's posi-

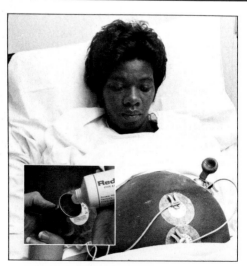

Using abdominal electrodes

Another way to monitor fetal heart rate (FHR) is by using an abdominal EKG monitor. Unlike the other FHR monitors, the abdominal EKG monitor also gives you a maternal-fetal EKG. Here's how it works.

In addition to a fetal monitor, you'll need alcohol swabs, electrode paste, two disposable abdominal electrodes, a suction electrode, and an electrode cable.

Using the first and second Leopold's maneuvers, determine the position of the fetus' head and back. If the fetus is in the left occiput anterior (LOA) position and is unengaged, the head and back will be in the lower left abdominal quadrant. Then follow these steps:
• Clean the selected sites on the mother's abdomen with the alcohol swabs, and allow the skin to dry.
• Gently abrade the skin at the selected sites, using the rough pad on the back of the electrodes. Then, apply the regular electrodes to the mother's abdomen, above the fetus' head and back.
• Place electrode paste inside the rim of the suction electrode (as shown in the inset).
• Apply the suction electrode over the fetus' buttocks. Note: If the fetus is in the LOA position, you'll locate its buttocks in the upper left abdominal quadrant.
• Attach the lead wire with the white clip to the electrode over the fetus' head. Then, attach the lead wire with the green clip to the electrode over the fetus' back.
• Finally, attach the lead wire with the black clip to the suction electrode. Your

heartbeat in the lower left quadrant of the mother's abdomen. The HEARTBEAT INDICATOR light on the monitor should flash with each audible heartbeat. The digital display will show the FHR. The FHR will also appear as a waveform on the oscilloscope screen.
• Secure the phonotransducer to the mother's abdomen with the belt, as the nurse is doing in the large photo to the left. But powder the belt first, so it's less irritating.
• Turn on the printout. This will give you the FHR waveform on printout paper. Determine if the tracing's adequate. If it isn't, reposition the phonotransducer and try again. Document what you've done in your nurses' notes.

tioned correctly? The HEARTBEAT light on the monitor flashes with every audible heartbeat. Take the mother's pulse as you watch the light. If her pulse corresponds with the flashing HEARTBEAT light, then you're not picking up the FHR; you're picking up uterine bruit, which corresponds to maternal pulse. To remedy this, adjust the position of the transducer.
• Slip the belt under the mother, and secure the transducer with it. But powder the belt first, to make it less irritating. Turn on the recorder printout. Make sure the FHR waveforms you're getting on the oscilloscope screen and on the recorder printout are acceptable.
At least once each hour during monitoring, reposition the transducer and carefully massage any red areas on the patient's skin. Then, wipe off excess jelly. This minimizes the risk of skin irritation.

setup should resemble the one in the large photo to the left.
• Plug the electrode cable into the EKG input on the fetal monitor. Depending on the doctor's orders, select either the EDIT or the UNEDIT mode. The EDIT mode averages every three heartbeats, while the UNEDIT mode lets every heartbeat be displayed on the oscilloscope screen and the printout.
• Turn on the monitor, and check the maternal-fetal EKG waveforms on the oscilloscope screen to make sure they're adequate. If you aren't getting a good signal, get new electrodes, and start the application procedure over. Check the digital display for FHR. To get FHR in printout form, turn on the printout.
Remember, document what you've done in your nurses' notes.

Nurses' guide to maternal-fetal EKGs

When you're monitoring with abdominal electrodes, how do you interpret maternal-fetal EKGs that appear on the oscilloscope screen? First, you must learn to distinguish between the maternal waveform and the fetal waveform, because the two appear on the screen together. The maternal heartbeat signal makes a tall, spiked waveform. The fetal heartbeat signal makes a waveform that's only a fraction of that size.

Second, you must know how to read the waveforms. You'll find that even an excellent quality signal won't yield a normal EKG pattern of P, QRS, and T waves. Therefore, you can't read a maternal EKG and a fetal EKG as easily as you'd read a normal EKG. In a maternal-fetal EKG, the important things to look for are consistency of the wave configurations and of the intervals between spikes.

Here are some examples of maternal-fetal EKG waveforms:

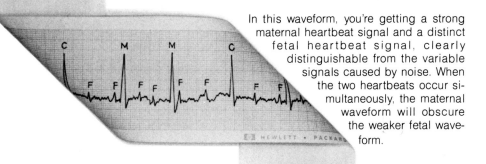

In this waveform, you're getting a strong maternal heartbeat signal and a distinct fetal heartbeat signal, clearly distinguishable from the variable signals caused by noise. When the two heartbeats occur simultaneously, the maternal waveform will obscure the weaker fetal waveform.

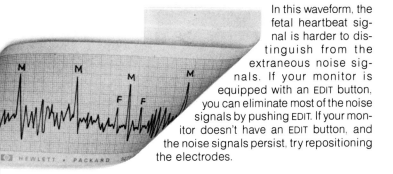

In this waveform, the fetal heartbeat signal is harder to distinguish from the extraneous noise signals. If your monitor is equipped with an EDIT button, you can eliminate most of the noise signals by pushing EDIT. If your monitor doesn't have an EDIT button, and the noise signals persist, try repositioning the electrodes.

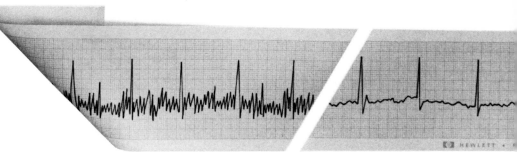

In this waveform, the fetal heartbeat signal is impossible to distinguish from the extraneous noise signals. If the distortion wasn't caused by a sudden movement of the mother, you may have to reposition the electrodes to get a better signal.

In this waveform, the fetal heartbeat signal is absent. If you can't locate a fetal heartbeat by repositioning the electrodes, notify the doctor. Then use a doptone to determine if the fetus is in distress or dead.

External fetal monitors

TROUBLESHOOTING

Troubleshooting inadequate uterine pressure waveforms

Problem	Possible causes	Solutions
Poor waveform or no waveform	• Uterine contractions not registering • Loose connection in equipment • Stylus not positioned correctly on printout paper	• Make sure the mother's positioned correctly. • Make sure the belt is tight and all connections are secure. • Adjust the position of stylus. • Make sure the pressure-sensitive button isn't impeded in any way: for example, from old jelly.
Abnormal-looking waveform or artifacts (waveform interference)	• Monitor improperly grounded • Fetal movement • Abnormal contractions	• Make sure you've grounded the monitor to a pipe or faucet. • Allow time for fetus to quiet down. If abnormal waveform persists, notify the doctor. • Observe the mother. When she changes position, coughs, or sneezes, note the activity on the printout paper.

Troubleshooting inadequate fetal heartbeat waveforms

Problem	Possible causes	Solutions
Poor waveform or no waveform	*When you're using any external fetal heart monitor:*	
	• Change in fetus' position, creating artifacts (waveform interference)	• Repeat the Leopold's maneuvers to reassess fetus' position. Allow time for the fetus to relax. Reposition transducer or electrodes, if necessary.
	• Malfunctioning equipment	• Consult operator's manual. Request repair service, if necessary.
	• Weak or unobtainable fetal heartbeat signal	• Make sure transducer or electrodes are firmly and properly placed. Check and secure connections. Use a fetoscope or doptone to scan all four quadrants of the uterus. If you still can't find a fetal heartbeat, notify the doctor. The fetus may be dead.
	When you're using an ultrasonic transducer or a phonotransducer only:	
	• Movement of mother during advanced labor	• Make sure belt is secure. Reposition transducer, if necessary.
	• Recording of blood flow through the placenta	• Readjust transducer angle for better quality recording.
	• Obese abdomen, making penetration difficult	• Reposition mother and/or transducer, as necessary. If you still can't get a good quality reading, consult the doctor about internal monitoring.
	When you're using an ultrasonic transducer or abdominal electrodes only:	
	• Dry or insufficient amount of contact jelly on electrodes or transducer	• Remove old contact jelly and apply new jelly. Repeat procedure every 2 hours, or as needed.

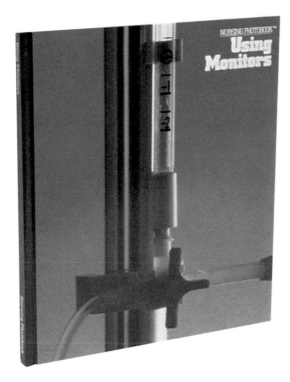

Ever get so wrapped up with equipment you almost forget your patient's there?

With *Using Monitors,* you'll learn to manage equipment *more confidently* so you can provide your patient with better care. You'll be amazed by how many new procedures and timesaving techniques you can quickly learn... at home!

So order your free 10-day examination copy of this PHOTOBOOK *today.*

Use or pass along this convenient order card.

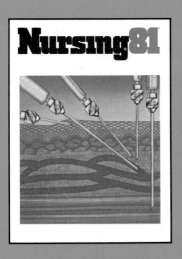

Get acquainted with the world's largest nursing journal today!

Using Monitors...your introduction to the brand-new NURSING PHOTOBOOK series

...the remarkable breakthrough in nursing education that can change your career. Each book in this unique series contains detailed *Photostories*... and tables, charts, and graphs to help you learn important new procedures. And each handsome PHOTOBOOK offers you • 160 illustrated, fact-filled pages • brilliant, high-contrast photographs • convenient 9"x10½" size • durable, hardcover binding • carefully chosen bibliography • complete index. Watch the experts at work showing you how to... administer drugs... teach your patient about his illness and its treatment... minimize trauma... understand doctors' diagnoses... increase patient comfort... and much more. Discover how you can become a better nurse by joining this exciting new series. You can examine each PHOTOBOOK at your leisure... for 10 days *absolutely free!*

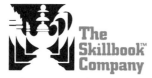
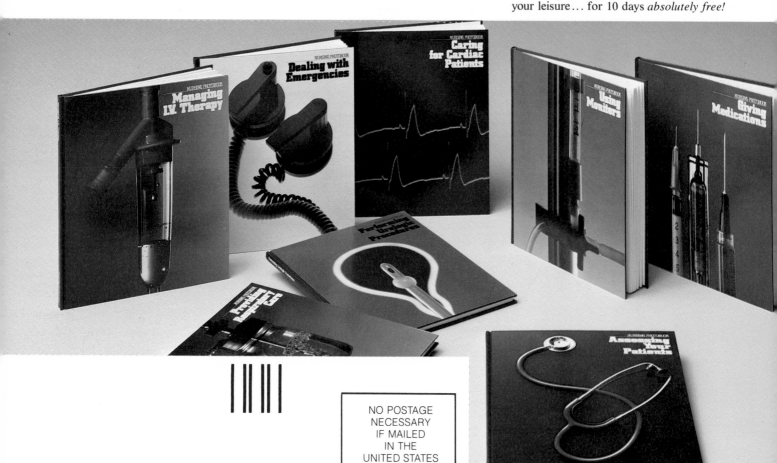

Be sure to mail the postage-paid card at left to reserve *your* first copy of *Nursing81!*

Internal fetal monitors

Your patient is in labor. During her last pregnancy, she developed uteroplacental insufficiency, which caused fetal hypoxia. Now, her doctor wants to make sure the health of this fetus won't be jeopardized like the last one. So, to help him tell if the fetus is in distress, he'll use a fetal scalp electrode and a uterine pressure catheter.

Want to learn about these pieces of equipment? How the doctor inserts them? How you should assist him? Then read the following pages. You'll learn all you need to know about internal fetal monitoring.

**Internal fetal monitoring:
Advantages and disadvantages**

Why use internal fetal monitoring when external monitoring is noninvasive and easier to initiate? Because internal monitoring doesn't pick up extraneous interference like external monitoring does. In advanced stages of labor, when the fetus has descended and the mother is changing her position frequently to minimize her discomfort, extraneous noise can become so great that an external monitoring printout is difficult to interpret. But internal monitoring picks up only the fetal heartbeat and the uterine contractions. The waveforms it produces are free of most interference and unaffected by maternal repositioning or fetal descent.

However, internal monitoring does have some drawbacks, which the doctor must consider. For example, a scalp electrode has the following disadvantages:
• It may cause abscesses or lacerations, with possible infection.
• It may cause fetal cerebral spinal fluid leakage, if placed in the fetus' scalp improperly.
• It can't be inserted into the fetus' face, if that's the presenting part.
A uterine catheter has these disadvantages:
• It can't be used in cases of maternal uterine infection, or placenta previa.
• It may perforate uterine lining, if improperly inserted.
• It may cause a prolapsed umbilical cord.
• It may cause eye injuries, if improperly placed.
• It may cause fetal distress, if improperly inserted.

Learning about internal monitors

How do the fetal scalp electrode and uterine pressure catheter work? Although both types of internal monitors operate on principles you've learned earlier in this book, the following information may help you understand them better.

• **Fetal scalp electrode:** A small corkscrew-type electrode that the doctor inserts in the presenting part of the fetus (unless it's the face). The electrode picks up the fetal heartbeat and transmits it to the monitor, which translates the impulse into a fetal EKG waveform on the oscilloscope screen and a fetal heart rate waveform on the printout. By observing and interpreting these waveforms, the doctor can tell immediately if the fetus' health is in jeopardy.

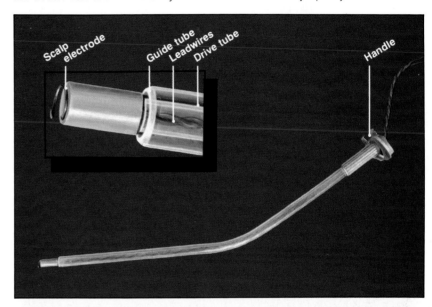

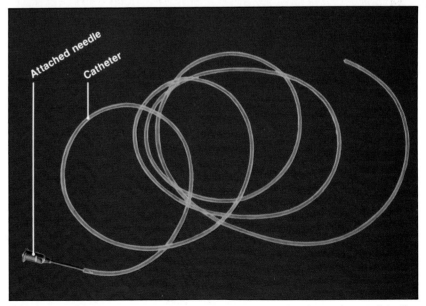

• **Uterine pressure catheter:** A fluid-filled tube that the doctor inserts into the uterus and connects to a pressure transducer and monitor. With each uterine contraction, fluid is displaced in the catheter, which in turn moves the diaphragm in the transducer. The transducer converts this pressure into an electrical impulse that's displayed in millimeters of mercury (mm Hg) on the monitor's screen. With this type of monitoring, the doctor can tell immediately when the mother's contractions become too weak or too strong for the fetus' well-being.

Internal fetal monitors

Helping to insert a fetal scalp electrode

Mrs. Roberta Torrence, a 32-year-old mother of two, is in advanced labor, and is about to give birth. Because she's had a history of complications during labor, her doctor wants to continuously monitor the fetal heartbeat. To do this, he'll have to insert a fetal scalp electrode (which can be used on any part of the fetus except its face). Here's how you'll assist him:

First, gather this equipment: fetal monitor, fetal scalp electrode, leg plate and attached cable, leg plate strap, and EKG paste.

Next, the doctor will perform a vaginal exam. Before he can continue the procedure, he must make sure the amniotic membrane is ruptured and the cervix dilated at least 2 cm. Then he'll identify the presenting part of the fetus. If it's something other than the fetus' face, he can begin inserting the scalp electrode immediately. However, if the presenting part is the fetus' face, the doctor won't insert the scalp electrode. He'll use the less precise external fetal EKG monitoring method instead.

As the illustration on the preceding page shows, the scalp electrode is mounted on the end of the drive tube, which is encased in the guide tube. Before he begins insertion, the doctor will make sure the electrode is retracted about 1" from the mouth of the guide tube. Then, he'll place the guide tube within the patient's cervix, firmly against the presenting part of the fetus, and advance the drive tube until he senses that the electrode's touching the fetus. When that's accomplished, he'll rotate the drive tube one turn clockwise or until he meets with mild resistance. This will insert the electrode into the fetus.

Next, he'll unlock the handle from the drive tube and remove it. Doing so will allow him to slip off the guide tube first, then the drive tube, leaving the scalp electrode in place and the entwined electrode wires exposed.

Now, the doctor will probably ask you to take over. Here's how:
• First, attach the electrode wires to their color-coded mates on the leg plate.
• Then, apply a generous coating of EKG paste to the underside of the plate. Place the plate on the patient's thigh.
• Use a leg plate strap to secure the plate to her thigh.
• Then, plug the leg plate cable into the monitor's EKG INPUT outlet, and press the monitor button marked POWER. This will cause the fetal EKG to appear on the oscilloscope screen.
• Finally, press the button marked RECORD to begin the printout of the fetal heart rate waveform.

Now the fetal EKG and heart rate can be monitored through the final stages of labor.

If the scalp electrode falls off, the doctor won't try to reinsert it, because that can cause an infection. Instead, he'll insert a new electrode.

What can you do if you're getting a poor EKG waveform? Take the following steps, in this order:
• Recheck electrodes to make sure they were applied and connected to the leg plate properly.
• Recheck the leg plate to make sure that it's been adequately secured to the mother's thigh and that it has enough electrode paste underneath it.
• Recheck leg plate cable connection to monitor.
• Make sure the monitor is working properly.
• Rule out fetal death using external monitoring.
• As a last resort, obtain a new scalp electrode. (The doctor will insert it.)

When labor's completed, the doctor will remove the scalp electrode from the newborn infant by simply turning the electrode counterclockwise until it comes loose. Clean the electrode's insertion site with betadine solution.

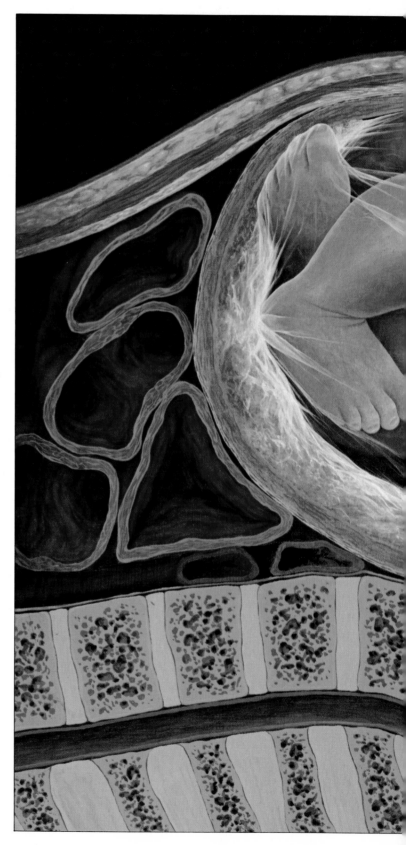

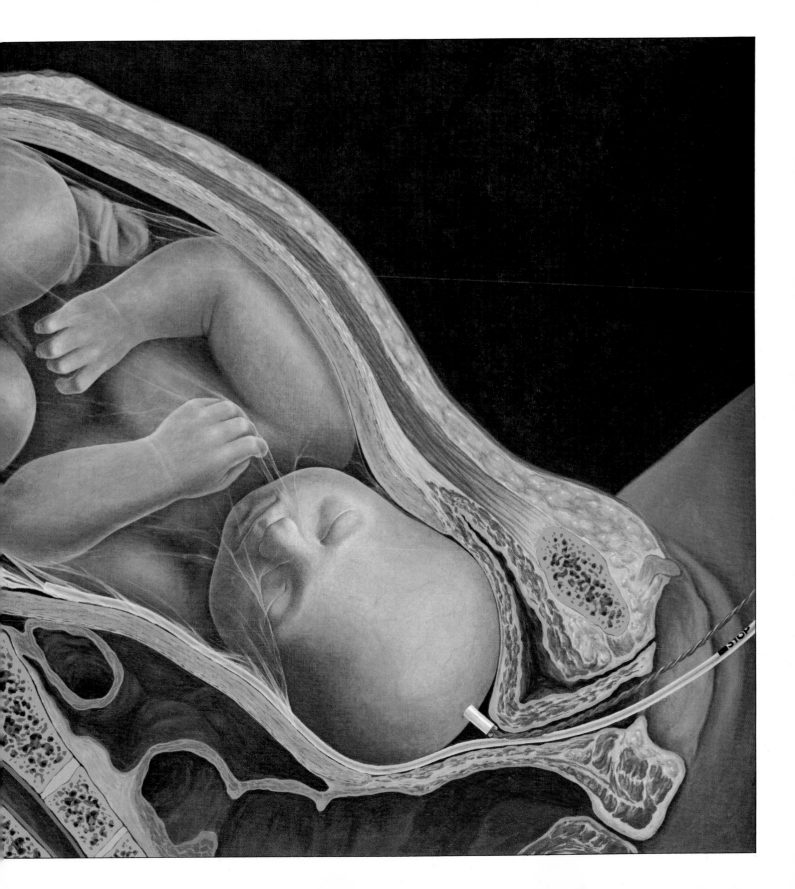

Internal fetal monitors

Helping initiate uterine pressure monitoring

1 *Mrs. Torrence is in the labor room. Her doctor has inserted a fetal scalp electrode and is monitoring the fetal heartbeat. He also wants to monitor her uterine pressure. Do you know how to prepare for uterine pressure monitoring?*

First, gather this equipment: a fetal monitor, nonallergenic tape, distilled water (all of which not shown), a transducer with a cable attached, a transducer dome, a pressure-release valve, a uterine catheter and guide tube with an I8G 1½" needle, a 20 cc syringe, a three-way stopcock, and a sterile glove.

2 Plug the transducer cable into the UTERINE ACTIVITY outlet on the monitor, as shown here. Then, plug the monitor into a standard wall outlet. Press the POWER button to turn the monitor on.

3 Now, place several drops of distilled water on the transducer diaphragm, and screw on the disposable plastic dome. Attach the pressure-release valve to the upright arm of the dome.

4 Attach the needle to the syringe and draw up 20 ml distilled water. Then, pick up the uterine catheter, which is encased inside the guide tube, and insert the syringe needle into it. Flush the catheter with 5 ml distilled water. Leave the syringe and needle attached to the catheter.

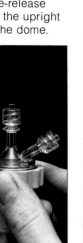

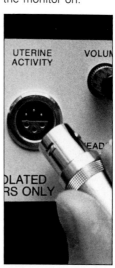

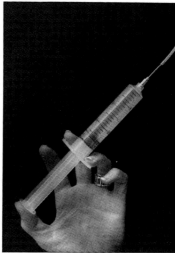

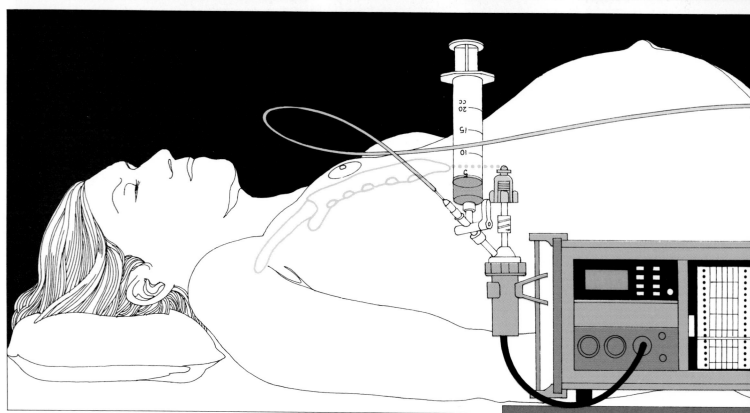

5 Attach a three-way stopcock to the sidearm on the transducer dome, while the doctor examines your patient vaginally. He'll want to make sure the uterine membrane's ruptured and the cervix dilated about 2 cm. Then, he'll insert the catheter and guide tube into the cervix. After he's inserted them, he'll advance the catheter (but not the guide tube) until the designated marker—usually the word STOP printed on the catheter—reaches the introitus. Then, he'll slide the guide tube up the catheter and away from the introitus. He'll probably ask you to secure the catheter to the mother's thigh. Do so, using nonallergenic tape.

6 Now, remove the syringe from the end of the inserted catheter, but leave the needle in place. Attach the needle hub to the lateral port of the three-way stopcock, as shown here.

7 Then, attach the syringe to the middle port of the three-way stopcock. Turn the stopcock lever so it's off to the transducer. Flush the catheter with 5 ml distilled water.

8 Now, rotate the stopcock lever so it's off to the patient. Lift the pressure-release valve with one hand, and using the syringe attached to the stopcock, inject water into the transducer dome to flush out any air bubbles. Remove the syringe to open the transducer to atmospheric pressure.

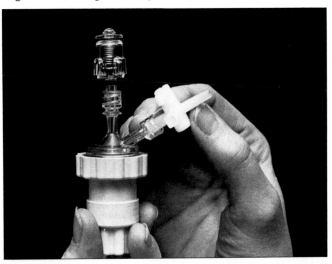
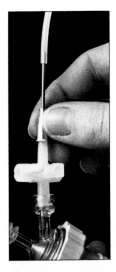
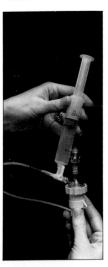
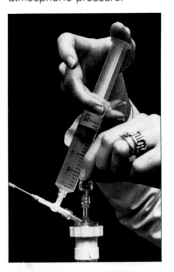

9 Now, mount the transducer onto the plastic clip on the side of the monitor. Level the pressure-release valve with the middle of your patient's uterus. To make sure you do, visualize a straight line extending from her xyphoid process down her side (see illustration). If you don't, you'll get false low readings by positioning the valve above the middle of her uterus and false high readings by positioning the valve below the middle of her uterus. Balance the transducer to atmospheric pressure, following the procedure described on page 15.

Replace the syringe on the open port, and turn the stopcock lever so it's off to the syringe. Expect to get a uterine pressure reading almost immediately. *Note:* The mother's contractions may increase in sensitivity to the point where

they force amniotic fluid through the catheter into the pressure-release valve. How can you tell? The valve will be moist. If this occurs, turn the stopcock lever so it's off to the patient. Then, lift the valve, and flush the dome and valve with 5 ml distilled water.

Suppose the uterine pressure readings damp during the monitoring process. Turn the stopcock lever off to the transducer, and flush the catheter with 5 ml distilled water. Then, turn the stopcock lever so it's closed to the syringe and open between the transducer and the patient.

During internal monitoring, the doctor will minimize the risk of infection by not conducting manual vaginal examinations unless absolutely necessary and by never monitoring for more than 8 hours at a time.

Internal fetal monitors

Troubleshooting uterine pressure monitoring

If the waveform on your uterine pressure monitor is too small to read, you may have one of the following problems:
• improper lever position on stopcock
• improper connection of catheter to stopcock
• improper leveling of transducer with maternal xyphoid process

• improper connections between transducer, cable, and monitor.

If you rule out all these problems and the waveform's still too small, you may have air bubbles or holes in the uterine catheter. If this is the case, the doctor will have to remove the catheter and replace it with a new one.

Monitoring the progress of the mother and fetus during labor

An internal fetal monitor can help you determine fetal well-being and maternal progress during labor. Consider the key to that determination the monitor printout. Here's what a typical internal fetal monitoring printout looks like:

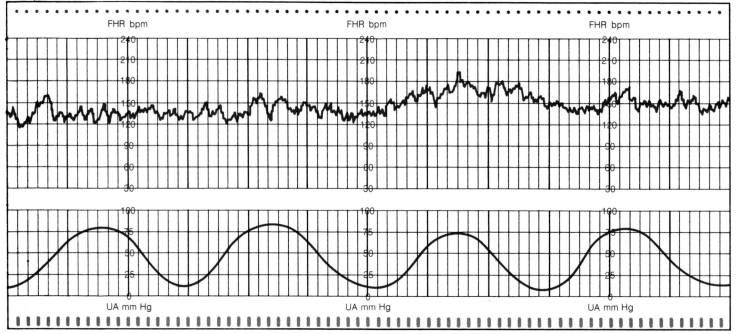

As you can see, it has two waveforms. The top waveform shows the fetal heart rate (not fetal EKG, which only appears on the oscilloscope screen). The bottom waveform shows the intensity, rate, and duration of uterine contractions. You'll want to compare the two after you interpret them individually.

First, interpret the fetal heart rate waveform, using the guidelines on pages 142 and 143. Determine both the baseline and the periodic heart rate. Then, interpret the uterine contraction waveform to determine the contraction's intensity, rate, and duration. How does this relate to cervical dilation? Study the chart to the right to know approximately what to expect.

Now, compare your fetal heart rate interpretation with your uterine contractions interpretation. Since contractions directly affect the fetal heart rate, this comparison will help you learn even more about the health of the fetus. Ask yourself these questions:
• What happens to the fetal heart rate when the mother has a normal contraction? Does it accelerate, decelerate, or stay the same?
• When the contraction ends, what happens to the fetal heart rate? Does it stay the same, return to normal, or slow to a dangerous level?
• As the contractions become more frequent and intense, how does

the fetal heart rate respond? Does it return to normal after each contraction or does it remain elevated?

Evaluate the waveforms about every 15 minutes. But do it more frequently if labor's being induced, if fetal heart rate changes dramatically, or if there's evidence of breech presentation (meconium staining).

Discuss your comparisons with the doctor. He'll use this information to determine how he'll manage the labor and birth.

Cervical dilation	Duration of contractions	Intensity of contractions	Frequency of contractions
1 to 2 cm	20 to 30 sec	30 to 50 mm Hg	6 to 8 min apart
2 to 4 cm	30 to 35 sec	50 to 75 mm Hg	5 to 6 min apart
4 to 6 cm	40 to 50 sec	50 to 75 mm Hg	4 to 5 min apart
6 to 8 cm	45 to 60 sec	50 to 75 mm Hg	3 to 4 min apart
8 to 10 cm	50 to 80 sec	50 to 75 mm Hg	2 to 3 min apart

Acknowledgements

**We'd like to thank
the following people
and companies for
their help with
this PHOTOBOOK:**

AMERICAN EDWARDS LABORATORIES
Critical Care Group
Irvine, Calif.

BELL & HOWELL
Medical Products
Van Nuys, Calif.
Carl M. Schuh,
Marketing Manager

COROMETRICS MEDICAL SYSTEMS, INC.
Wallingford, Conn.
Timothy Murphy,
Sales Consultant

EforM/HONEYWELL INC.
Boothwyn, Pa.
Guy Capone,
Regional Manager

GOULD, INC.
Medical Products Division
Oxnard, Calif.

HEALTHCO, INC.
Reading, Pa.
Al Szymborski, CMR

HEWLETT-PACKARD
Waltham, Mass.
Maryanne Schreiber, RN,
Marketing Specialist

LADD RESEARCH INDUSTRIES, INC.
Burlington, Vt.
Margaret W. Ladd,
President
John Arnott,
Director of Marketing

Fred Letterio,
Medical Instrumentation Specialist
University of Pennsylvania
Philadelphia, Pa.

MEDICAL MONITORS, INC.
Wyncote, Pa.
Michael Pennock, President

Donald L. Myers, MD,
Clinical Instructor, Neurosurgical
Thomas Jefferson University Hospital
Philadelphia, Pa.

NARCO AIR-SHIELDS, INC.
Division of NARCO Scientific
Hatboro, Pa.

ROCHE MEDICAL ELECTRONICS INC.
Cranbury, N.J.

SORENSON RESEARCH COMPANY
Salt Lake City, Utah
R. James Jones,
Eastern Zone Manager
Rae Nadine Smith, RN, MS,
Clinical Nursing Specialist

Also the staffs of:

ALBERT EINSTEIN MEDICAL CENTER
Philadelphia, Pa.

DELAWARE VALLEY MEDICAL CENTER
Bristol, Pa.

PENNSYLVANIA HOSPITAL
Philadelphia, Pa.

THOMAS JEFFERSON UNIVERSITY HOSPITAL
Philadelphia, Pa.

Suggested further reading

Books

Andreoli, Kathleen, et al. COMPREHENSIVE CARDIAC CARE, 4th ed. St. Louis: C.V. Mosby Co., 1979.

Avery Mary E., and Barry D. Fletcher. THE LUNG AND ITS DISORDERS IN THE NEWBORN INFANT, 3rd ed. Philadelphia: W.B. Saunders Co., 1974.

Berne, Robert M., and Matthew N. Levy. CARDIOVASCULAR PHYSIOLOGY, 3rd ed. St. Louis: C.V. Mosby Co., 1977.

Boscala, M., et al. CLINICAL ELEMENTS OF FETAL HEART RATE MONITORING. Waltham, Mass.: Hewlett-Packard, 1977.

Brehm, J.J., et al. THE HEART, ARTERIES AND VEINS. New York: McGraw-Hill Book Co., 1978.

Bruce, Derek A. THE PATHOPHYSIOLOGY OF INCREASED INTRACRANIAL PRESSURE. Kalamazoo, Mich.: Upjohn Co., 1978.

Burton, George, et al. RESPIRATORY CARE. Philadelphia: J.B. Lippincott Co., 1977.

Clark, Ann L., and Dyanne D. Affonso. CHILDBEARING: A NURSING PERSPECTIVE, 2nd ed. Philadelphia: F.A. Davis Co., 1979.

COPING WITH NEUROLOGIC PROBLEMS PROFICIENTLY. *Nursing* Skillbook®. Horsham, Pa.: Intermed Communications, Inc., 1979.

GUIDE TO PHYSIOLOGIC MONITORING. Waltham, Mass.: Hewlett-Packard Co., 1977.

Guyton, A.C. TEXTBOOK OF MEDICAL PHYSIOLOGY, 5th ed. Philadelphia: W.B. Saunders Co., 1976.

Hill, D.W., and A.M. Dolan. INSTRUMENTATION FOR INTENSIVE CARE. New York: Grune & Stratton, 1976.

Holloway, Nancy M. NURSING THE CRITICALLY ILL ADULT. Reading, Mass.: Addison-Wesley Pub. Co., 1979.

Hudak, Carolyn M. CRITICAL CARE NURSING, 2nd ed. Philadelphia: J.B. Lippincott Co., 1977.

Hurst, J. Willis. THE HEART. New York: McGraw-Hill Book Co., 1978.

INSTRUCTION MANUAL—CARDIAC OUTPUT COMPUTER. Ervine, Calif.: American Edwards Laboratories.

MANAGING I.V. THERAPY. *Nursing* PHOTOBOOK™ Series. Horsham, Pa.: Intermed Communications, Inc., 1980.

MANUAL FOR RE 134 RESPIRATION MODULE. Fort Worth, Tex.: Electronic Monitors, Inc.

Meltzer, Lawrence, et al. INTENSIVE CORONARY CARE, 3rd ed. Bowie, Md.: Charles Press Publishers, 1977.

Miller, S., et al. METHODS IN CRITICAL-CARE—THE A.A.C.N. MANUAL. Philadelphia: W.B. Saunders Co., 1980.

NURSING CRITICALLY ILL PATIENTS CONFIDENTLY. *Nursing* Skillbook®. Horsham, Pa.: Intermed Communications, Inc., 1979.

READING EKGs CORRECTLY. *Nursing* Skillbook®. Horsham, Pa.: Intermed Communications, Inc., 1975.

Schroeder, John S., and Elaine K. Daily. TECHNIQUES IN BEDSIDE HEMODYNAMIC MONITORING, 2nd ed. St. Louis: C.V. Mosby Co., 1980.

Tucker, S. FETAL MONITORING AND FETAL ASSESSMENT IN HIGH-RISK PREGNANCY. St. Louis: C.V. Mosby Co., 1978.

Webb, W.R. LUNG PERFUSION AND OXYGEN UPTAKE. Monograph in THE ORGAN IN SHOCK, Proceedings of the second symposium on recent research development and current clinical practice in shock, 1977.

Wilson, Robert Francis, ed. PRINCIPLES AND TECHNIQUES OF CRITICAL CARE. Kalamazoo, Mich.: Upjohn Co., 1976.

Periodicals

Boehm, F.H. *FHR Variability: Key to Fetal Well-Being,* CONTEMPORARY OB/GYN. May 1977.

Bonner, John T. *Clinical Use of the Pulmonary Artery (Swan-Ganz) Catheter,* ANESTHESIOLOGY REVIEW. July 1977.

Dulock, H.J., and M. Herron. *Women's Response to Fetal Monitoring,* JOURNAL OF OBSTETRICS, GYNECOLOGY, AND NEONATAL NURSING. September-October 1976.

Eccles, Lynn, and Barbara Stranger. *Intracranial Pressure Monitoring: The Swollen Brain,* LIFE SUPPORT NURSING. January-February 1980.

Evaluation—Blood Pressure Monitors, HEALTH DEVICES. November 1975.

Fisher, Ruth E. *Measuring Central Venous Pressure: How to Do It Accurately... and Safely,* NURSING79. 9:74-78, October 1979.

Gingerich, B., and C. Martin. *Uteroplacental Physiology,* JOURNAL OF OBSTETRICS, GYNECOLOGY, AND NEONATAL NURSING. 5:16-25, September-October 1976.

Goodlin, R. *History of Fetal Monitoring,* AMERICAN JOURNAL OF OBSTETRICS AND GYNECOLOGY. 133:327-347, February 1979.

Hanlon, Kathryn. *Description and Uses of Intra-Cranial Pressure Monitoring,* HEART & LUNG. 5:277-282, March-April 1976.

Horovitz, J.W., and A. Leterman. *Postoperative Monitoring Following Critical Trauma,* HEART & LUNG. 4:270, 1975.

The Infection Hazards of Pressure Monitoring Devices, C.D.C. NATIONAL NOSOCOMIAL INFECTION STUDY REPORT. April 1977.

Jennings, B.M., and E.H. Niggemann. *Use of Balloon-tipped Flow-directed Catheter to Assess Pulmonary Status,* CRITICAL CARE QUARTERLY. 2:11-13, 1979.

Lalli, Susan M. *The Complete Swan-Ganz,* RN. September 1978.

Lamb J. *Intra-Arterial Monitoring: Rescinding the Risks,* NURSING77. 7:65-68, November 1977.

Left Atrial Pressure Lines, I.C.U. POLICY AND PROCEDURE MANUAL. Albert Einstein Medical Center, Northern Division, Philadelphia, 1978.

Levin, Allan B. *The Use of a Fiberoptic Pressure Transducer in the Treatment of Head Injuries,* THE JOURNAL OF TRAUMA. 17:767-774, October 1977.

Lowenshohn, R. *Instrumentation for Fetal Heart Rate Monitoring,* JOURNAL OF OBSTETRICS, GYNECOLOGY, AND NEONATAL NURSING. 5:7-10, September-October 1976.

Melville, A., et al. *Fetal Heart Rate Accelerations in Labor: Excellent Prognostic Indicator,* AMERICAN JOURNAL OF OBSTETRICS AND GYNECOLOGY. 134:36-38, May 1979.

Mitchell, Pamela H., and Nancy Mauss. *Intracranial Pressure: Fact and Fancy,* NURSING76. 6:53-57, June 1976.

Nichols, Wilmer W., et al. *Complications Associated with Balloon-tipped, Flow-directed Catheters,* HEART & LUNG. 8:503-506, May-June 1979.

Nielsen, M. *Arterial Monitoring of Blood Pressure,* AMERICAN JOURNAL OF NURSING. 74:48, January 1974.

Nikas, Diane, and Rose Konkoly. *Nursing Responsibilities in Arterial and Intracranial Pressure Monitoring,* JOURNAL OF NEUROSURGICAL NURSING. 7:116-122, December 1975.

Respiration Modules, TECHNICAL DATA. Series 427 and 803. Mennen Medical Inc., Clarance, N.Y.

Schifrin, B. *The Rationale for Antepartum Fetal Heart Monitoring,* JOURNAL OF REPRODUCTIVE MEDICINE. 23:213-221, November 1979.

Sears, Martin F., and Charles Heise. *Troubleshooting the Swan-Ganz Catheter,* HEART & LUNG. 9:303-305, March-April 1980.

Smith, Rae N. *Invasive Pressure Monitoring,* AMERICAN JOURNAL OF NURSING. 78:1514-1521, September 1978.

Swanbrow, Diane. *The Rise of Mass Spectrometry in Respiratory Monitoring,* RESPIRATORY THERAPY. July-August 1978.

Swan-Ganz, Flow-directed Catheters, PRODUCT BULLETIN. American Edwards Laboratories, March 1979.

Turner, Michael. *Intracranial Hypertension,* CRITICAL CARE QUARTERLY. 2:67-76, 1979.

Vries, J.K., et al. *Subarachnoid Screw for Monitoring Intracranial Pressure,* JOURNAL OF NEUROSURGERY. 39:416-419, September 1973.

Walinsky, Paul. *Acute Hemodynamic Monitoring,* HEART & LUNG. 6:838-843, September-October 1977.

Woods, Susan L. *Monitoring Pulmonary Artery Pressures,* AMERICAN JOURNAL OF NURSING. 76:1765-1771, November 1976.

Index

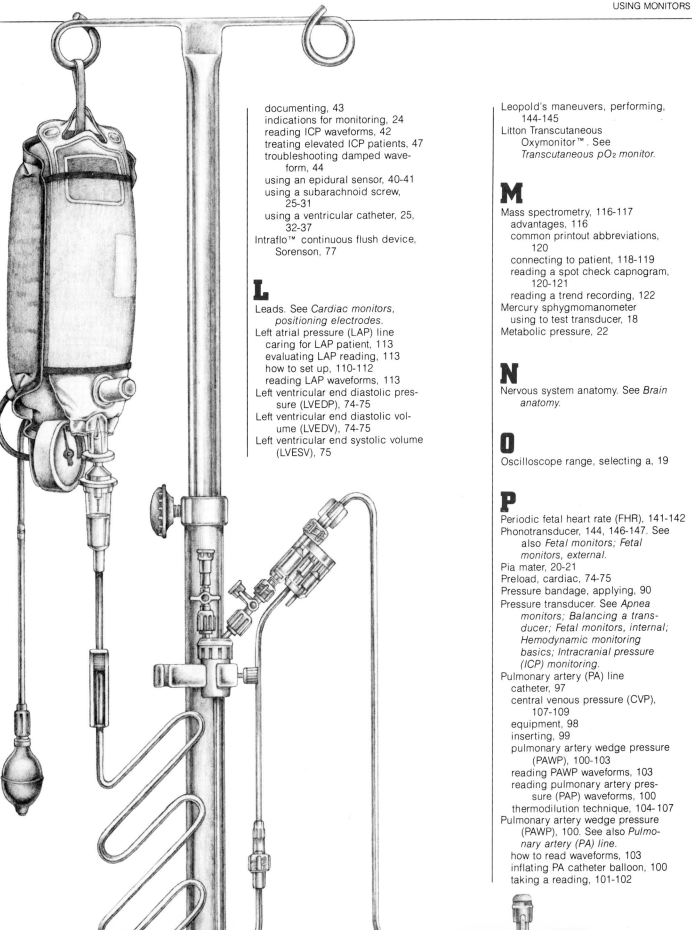

Index

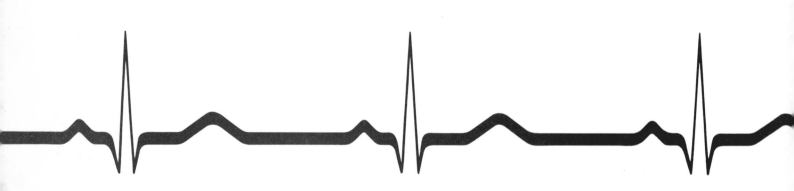